Praise for the Growing G.R.E.E.N. InterActions Program®

From a teacher:

The Growing G.R.E.E.N. InterActions program provides students with the opportunity to develop perspective-taking skills and to practice prosocial responses through role-play activities. The students in my class really enjoy the feeling of acting on stage. There are roles for everyone, including being the director, scene writers, movie characters, and audience members. The role-play activities provide students with the opportunity to practice new coping skills in a safe environment. There is nothing more enjoyable than to hear a student learn to use a response during the Growing G.R.E.E.N. InterActions program and generalize it to a situation.

Rosanne Lewton, Special Education Teacher

From a cotreating occupational therapist:

It has truly been a pleasure to have a collaborative relationship with Herb as he developed the G.R.E.E.N. approach. It has been enjoyable to watch the children learn and implement an approach that allows for proper expression of complex relation building ideas. The concepts and tools developed created a common language for all children and adults that opened successful positive communication where once there was an environment of closed and negative thoughts.

Mark Wilson, OTR, Occupational Therapist

From a cotreating counselor:

Working with Herb on Growing G.R.E.E.N. InterActions in the classroom was a fun and interactive way to teach our students about social skills and social communication. His approach to social communication is very helpful for all students regardless of primary diagnosis (i.e., ASD, ADHD, PTSD, Mood Disorder, ODD, etc.). Growing G.R.E.E.N. InterActions approaches communication using a framework from Cognitive Behavioral Therapy. It helps the student understand the processes behind specific interactions and the reasons why talking about the feelings of yourself and the feelings of others is important. It teaches kids how our behaviors do impact and affect the feelings, thoughts, and actions of those around us. Herb's approach is to help the students understand that everyone works as a team and how we affect one another. I think this is a much-needed aspect of social skills training. I highly recommend that SLPs, counselors, social workers, OTs, teachers and therapists use his curriculum in any school across the world.

Arielle Lugn, MA, PPS

Growing GREEN InterActions—*The Guide's Guide*

A Social Literacy Program to Be Our Better Selves in a Better World

Herb Hein, MMSc, CCC-SLP

Hein SLP, Inc. San Diego, California

Growing GREEN InterActions—*The Guide's Guide*

A Social Literacy Program to Be Our Better Selves in a Better World

Published by Hein SLP, Inc. San Diego, California

www.HeinSLPinc.com

Permissions, requests, and correspondence should be directed to the publisher.

ISBN-13: 978-0-9659878-0-6

This first edition printed in the United States of America.

Contents

Figures

Preface—Why and How This Program Was Developed

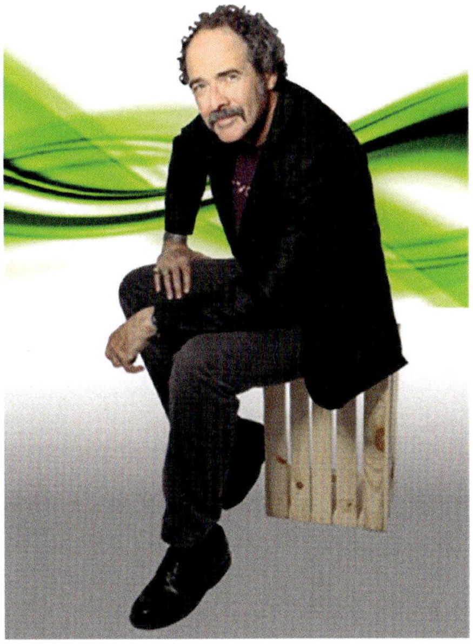

Herb Hein, MMSc, CCC-SLP

Growing G.R.E.E.N. InterActions® is the program I developed to improve the social skills of my clients and students. It also is the philosophy guiding my life and the choices I make in my daily interactions with others on my Teams—I navigate the scenes of my life using the program's guidelines, scripts, and guiding thoughts.

Often in our modern civilization, too little emphasis is placed on the best ways to communicate with others. The word Team stresses a critical component of the program—helping participants act more prosocial. Being with others is equivalent to being on their Teams, creating an opportunity to act in a prosocial, G.R.E.E.N. manner for the mutual benefit of Team members. Our society becomes better when we interact with others as if we are all on the same Team.

What guidelines should we follow to get along better with others in the same classroom, house, playground, workspace, and country? Are we

- following the basic social rules that people use when we enter a room?
- learning how to navigate a difference of opinion or point of view?
- learning strategies for coping with change or knowing what to do when others tell us "no"?
- learning how to negotiate and compromise?

These materials have helped my clients and students learn to share this G.R.E.E.N. philosophy and use it when taking action with others on their Teams.

Another central lesson of the program is that we all are responsible for making our experiences with other people better rather than worse. With the gift of our human brains, we have the power to choose to make things better for ourselves and those around us. We also can benefit from guidance in (1) making choices of how to act and (2) knowing what to say in different situations. It is my hope that this program will help you guide participants to feel more comfortable, skilled, and powerful when choosing actions to better their situations.

These materials were developed over several years working with students in private schools who exhibited language disorders, social–pragmatic challenges, and high-level autism. I further honed the materials while improving social language skills at the San Diego Center for Children Academy, a school for those struggling with emotional challenges. I was fortunate to present the G.R.E.E.N. InterActions materials and concepts as part of whole-class lessons for the school's elementary and middle school students. With everyone in these grades guided to speak the same "language" and receiving reinforcement for acting G.R.E.E.N., the change in the school's environment and culture was palpable. Students knew that everyone was working to show G.R.E.E.N. actions for their Class, School, and Friendship Teams. The school's students and staff made a more concerted effort to demonstrate G.R.E.E.N. actions to one another.

Being on the same Team increased participants' sense of unity because the language related to being on Teams was used in numerous daily interactions around campus:

- What is our Common Team Goal right now, and what are we doing to achieve it?
- What choices can we make now to help our Team?
- What G.R.E.E.N. action did you take to make our scene better?
- How can we act and what can we say to one another that shows we are Grateful, Respectful, Empathetic, and Easygoing?
- What Guiding G.R.E.E.N. Thought® did you use to Navigate that challenging situation?
- Let's act G.R.E.E.N. for the Team!

Students already at the Academy demonstrated to new students what acting G.R.E.E.N. means. The program's powerful, positive effects motivated me to expand the program in my private practice and ongoing consultations with schools and clinics.

I have helped people suffering from brain injuries and other neurological impairments to select personal goals that allowed them to monitor how well they paid attention to their environments and determined the actions to take. Clients work harder when goals are clearly delineated and presented for their review. Those with neurological and emotional impairments have found goal setting important for developing social skills and for overall emotional recovery. This can be achieved by discussing, setting, and visually displaying goals. Neurologically impaired adults find printed cues and verbal mediation strategies helpful for remembering tasks and guiding behaviors. This important focus on the value of goal-setting has been integrated into the Growing G.R.E.E.N. InterActions Program.

Printed cues and verbal mediation strategies were equally effective when guiding the social skills of those with high-level autism and emotional disturbance. The program's guiding strategies have also benefited participants in the general population for whom awareness of others and consideration of them when taking actions can only be learned by direct instruction.

During my career, I have worked with clients of every age, and I've had success treating a variety of disorders, but historically I was less comfortable working with emotionally disturbed individuals. Fortunately, at the time I started working at the San Diego Center for Children Academy, Ross Greene, PhD, presented a program that familiarized me with his effective approaches for working with "The Explosive Child" whose behaviors proved difficult to change. Reviewing his work made it possible for me to feel successful in working with this challenging population. I then developed my own speech-language pathology program to address the needs and goals for this population at the school in individual, small-group, and whole-class settings.

Among many extremely useful concepts, Dr. Greene stressed that some students were "lagging," displaying lower developmental levels in some basic skills that affected their interactions with others. This idea counteracted the thought that these students were just willfully choosing to act in maladaptive ways. The more hopeful, proactive concept was that with direct instruction of fundamental skills at early developmental levels, these students could learn to act differently. I developed materials to support development of the receptive, expressive, and social language skills necessary for participants to survey and analyze the social scene around them in order to choose the best prosocial action to benefit their Classroom, Home, and Friendship Teams. Some professionals I worked with doubted that students could understand the vocabulary related to these choices and the reasons why these choices were better, but after this program was implemented in several classrooms, it became apparent to these initial skeptics that through explicit instruction and numerous opportunities to practice prosocial actions and scenes, students understood what was presented, displaying this through positive changes in behavior.

Students with lagging language skills who participated in the program learned to assert themselves in expressing their feelings and what they needed. They learned vocabulary and language for better understanding their social challenges. This led to increased self-awareness and subsequently self-control. Through the practice of several scenes targeting needed behaviors, they improved their ability to say or do what would be considered prosocial and G.R.E.E.N. with gradually less cuing. It was extraordinary to observe them demonstrating that they cared by making a situation better rather than worse.

Students in the program realized that an effective dialogue was needed for accurately perceiving problems of the moment and determining what affected people could do about them. They recognized the need for Cooperative Conversations. I started working with the idea that teachers, parents, and students are on the same Team, thus allowing for a greater likelihood of more collaborative interactions. Both sides could be heard and acknowledged and a joint solution determined. I generated dialogues that included some key concepts that Ross Greene had shared, and developed these into interactions that highlighted proactive and mutually respectful behavior. I considered that any time a conversation occurred, there was also a Team. "What are we both trying to accomplish here in this scene?" Using language like this made students less defensive and allowed the staff to see that collaborative conversations were possible. I generated a framework for this, including scenes and scripts that helped participants engage more frequently in this cooperative, mutually beneficial mode of communicating. An additional focus was on developing participant awareness that scenes typically have more than one point of view, and this awareness of points of view and attempts to understand other points of view are critical for successful, cooperative interactions. Students were given opportunities to practice speaking in a more collaborative way, and teachers were provided with models in G.R.E.E.N. Scenes that spelled out what they could say to also be perceived as more collaborative. If you have not already done so, I suggest you read Ross W. Greene's book *The Explosive Child* and discover more of his collaborative problem-solving approach and his suggestions for assessing and treating this challenged population.

In my 40 years of clinical practice, I have learned the value of strong collaboration, cotreatment, and coteaching with other professionals. When developing this program, I worked closely with teachers who shared their classes with me. They contributed what they saw as the most prevalent social challenges that students experienced in their classrooms. I then wrote related material to help students analyze what was happening in those challenging social situations. Students used these materials and found examples of unhelpful, antisocial (R.E.D.) behavior. They were guided to see how such behavior negatively affected the rest of the Class Team and interfered with its attainment of the Common Team Goal of having a safe, respectful, and cooperative classroom where everyone could learn. Students were given materials to help them further develop the same social literacy skills for their Home Teams.

Their improved social literacy positively affected their Home Teams and enabled them to live in more peaceful, collaborative environments.

Students were given *explicit* instruction to replace unhelpful behavior with prosocial—G.R.E.E.N.—behavior. They were presented with scripts of exactly what to say and scenes where they could *frequently* practice using prosocial words in conversations. They experienced positive reinforcement from having made better action choices in the scenes. After students were given ideas of positive language that would fit a scene, some of the more verbal students formulated scripts to make their own scenes G.R.E.E.N. This motivated them to use prosocial approaches in their real-life scenes. The Growing G.R.E.E.N. InterActions Program includes complete scripts and structured opportunities for students to write their own prosocial dialogues.

It was amazing to see students who had rarely exhibited prosocial behavior eagerly acting out G.R.E.E.N. Scenes and exhibiting socially positive behaviors spontaneously! Though many professionals believed that these students were unwilling or unable to display prosocial behavior, many students displayed G.R.E.E.N. actions when they began to use G.R.E.E.N. language and better understood why improved action choices benefited the Team. When teachers, therapists, and I witnessed these dramatic transformations, I was motivated to turn these materials into a program that could be shared with others who could then experience the same powerful transformations with their students and clients.

Self-calming strategies were integrated into this program to support the occupational-therapy and speech-language goals of students. For example, the song "Brake to Take a Five Break" guides a self-calming, controlled breathing exercise, which a participant can be cued to use prior to the next step of choosing a prosocial action.

While implementing this program, I discovered that using its strategies myself assisted me in attaining and maintaining better relationships with others: my wife, children, students, and clients, their parents, and their spouses. It also helped me maintain relationships with those in the community who did not appear Grateful, Respectful, Empathetic, Easygoing, and Navigating. It is critical that one is extremely patient and acting G.R.E.E.N. when guiding participants to make prosocial G.R.E.E.N. choices, especially for participants who have not made such choices previously. This program helped me develop patience in situations where it had not come easily in the past.

I would be remiss if I did not mention how I have been encouraged to move forward with the development of my own transformative program by reading *Buddha's Brain: The Practical*

Neuroscience of Happiness, Love & Wisdom. This book by Rick Hanson, PhD, neuropsychologist, and meditation teacher, and Richard Mendius, MD and neurologist, is filled with neuroscientific research and practical suggestions that support and expound the idea that the brain can be rewired by experiencing more positive interactions and emotions. Our lives can be better when we are guided to think about our action choices. Our brains remain open to change throughout our life-spans:

> *How we focus our attention, how we intentionally direct the flow of energy and information through our neural circuits, can directly alter the brain's activity and its structure . . . the way we communicate alters the very circuitry of our brain, especially in ways that help keep our lives in balance.*[1]

Practicing Thinking First and using prosocial thoughts and scripts with the others around us positively affects the structure of our brains to make it easier to improve our neurological and social connections. I encourage you to read this book for its transformative recommendations, exercises, and related brain science explaining the power of our thoughts and actions.

Twenty years ago, I developed exercises that I published as *Strategy Power: Functional Listening Exercises* from working with brain-injured clients who needed to develop the power of assertive listening skills to compensate for memory and comprehension deficits. Hundreds of therapists and teachers around the country used that book to teach clients and students with varying degrees of listening impairments that arose from various disorders how to use assertive listening skills in the home, community, and workplace.

Now, I hope I have effectively shared with you how my newest program, Growing G.R.E.E.N. InterActions, has positively affected the students whom I have recently guided to develop broader sets of skills by learning to interact prosocially with others. I also hope you can see how my program aligns with existing treatment paradigms in related fields. Perhaps you are now inspired to take the next step and become a guide of the Growing G.R.E.E.N. InterActions Program—*The Guide's Guide* will assist you in such an endeavor.

Herb Hein, MMSc, CCC-SLP

Summer 2018

1. Buddha's Brain: The Practical Neuroscience of Happiness, Love & Wisdom. Rick Hanson, PhD and Richard Mendius, MD. New Harbinger Publications, Inc., 2009.

Acknowledgments

There are so many people to thank for helping the Growing G.R.E.E.N. InterActions Program become a reality. Numerous students of the San Diego Center for Children Academy were the first to be guided and motivated to "Act G.R.E.E.N. for the Team" through the lessons and activities I presented. It was a joy to see the pride in their faces as they successfully engaged in scripted and self-guided interactions. Their subsequent growth in social literacy motivated me to turn this into a program that could be used by other schools and programs throughout the country. Rosanne Lewton, Jim Mcelroy, Diana Brown, Jennifer Szwarc, and Stacey Gubens are elementary and middle school teachers who helped develop this program. They welcomed me into their classrooms for weekly G.R.E.E.N. lessons so we could collaborate together and improve the social skills of their students. I am indebted to Nancy Macnamara, the principal of the SDCC Academy, for supporting my innovation as I developed these lessons and activities.

I will always be extremely grateful for the opportunity to collaborate with Mark Wilson, an effective occupational therapist with whom I witnessed many positive changes in student behavior as we used these activities and G.R.E.E.N. Scenes in our co-led small OT and speech groups. Mark utilized strategies to increase participants' awareness of their feelings and incorporated strategies that participants could use to become calmer and more focused. While Mark worked to increase a student's self-calming ability using sensory-based strategies, I taught the student to understand and use words and scripts for choosing prosocial actions with increased independence.

I also have tremendous gratitude for school counselor Arielle Lugn, MA, PPS, a dynamic professional with whom I co-led lessons and witnessed remarkable growth in student social behavior. Arielle helped me understand the behavioral issues of students who were not on my speech-language caseload so that we could address the needs of everyone in each classroom. I appreciate that while using the concepts and language of this program, she confirmed its powerful cognitive–behavioral aspects. She helped support these cognitive–behavioral concepts by explaining to students how thoughts, feelings, and behavior interact.

I would also like to thank Sara Keepper, teacher of the Community Based Instruction Class of Grossmont Union High School District, with whom I have collaborated in using the Growing

G.R.E.E.N. InterActions Program with one of her autistic students. These materials have significantly developed this young adult student's ability to interact more appropriately with her Home, School, and Work Teams. Thanks go to the clients within my private practice and their parents with whom I used this program. I am grateful these families could work together in my office and in their homes to improve the interactions of their Home Teams.

Thank you to Marlene Beard, Alma Gutierrez, Kim Romano and Janis Wohlford, the office managers of Hein Speech-Language Pathology, Inc., who helped me organize and lay out all of the material in the different evolutionary phases. Thank you also to Heidi Utley, who spent weekly meetings during the year between her undergraduate and graduate programs in speech-language pathology to review and discuss initial drafts of the *Interactive Lesson Book* and *Guide's Guide*. I am also grateful for the time spent by colleagues who reviewed the program to provide me with useful feedback: Ingrid Exerjian and Mindy Mattison, both speech-language pathologists, and Sue Geller, elementary school principal.

Thank you to Jeff Berkley, who produced, recorded, and mixed the music on *Songs for Guiding G.R.E.E.N. Thoughts*. I initially wrote and played the songs, but he chose the musicians and backup singers that made each individual song more powerful. Thanks to all those incredible musicians and singers, including my musical partner, Jeff Proctor. Thank you also to Jordan Morita for the musical transcriptions for each of the songs. Thanks also go to my brother, Rick Hein, for encouraging me to write the "Guiding G.R.E.E.N. Thought Song."

Thank you to the graphic artists involved in this program, Micah Cerelli, and my daughter, Natalie Hein. They produced the icons and illustrations that I was visualizing in my mind so that I could successfully depict the key concepts of this program. Thank you to my son, Adam Hein, for sharing his photographic and video talents to support my work. Thank you to Amy Stanko, of Pixel Lava Interactive, the designer who brought new life to our website so we could more effectively share with those people interested in the program. Thank you to Brent Tharp, managing editor of Atlas Publishing, for guiding the format of *The Growing G.R.E.E.N. InterActions Lesson Book* and *The Guide's Guide* so that they can be in the hands of those who can benefit from them.

Gratitude beyond words goes to my wife and business partner in our speech-language pathology private practice, Joanne Gerstein Hein, who provided the encouragement throughout the six years that it took to get this program developed and published. As the first editor, she took the time to read every word and provide invaluable feedback along the way.

I am particularly grateful for the love and support from my children, Adam and Natalie Hein, and my wife, Joanne. These are the people who have inspired and encouraged my music and creative thoughts. These are the cherished people with whom I have built a Team, and it is through the growth of our own G.R.E.E.N. interactions that I realize the true value of this program. I look forward to interacting and making our best choices together as our family grows in the future.

Thank you also to my parents, Bernard and Lillian Hein, who guided me from above while I worked on developing this program, to make the most of my life by engaging in projects that would be meaningful and beneficial to others.

Herb Hein, MMSc, CCC-SLP

Summer 2018

1 Introduction

Welcome to ***The Guide's Guide*** for **Growing G.R.E.E.N. InterActions**!

The Guide's Guide is intended for teachers, therapists, and parents who will guide participants journeying through the **Growing G.R.E.E.N. InterActions Program**®. This guidebook explains the program's purpose and how to best use the materials presented. In this way, both guides and participants can see improvements in social functioning, first in structured activities and then in real-life situations. Through your guidance, others will learn the skills needed to act increasingly more G.R.E.E.N.: Grateful, Respectful, Empathetic, Easygoing, and Navigating.

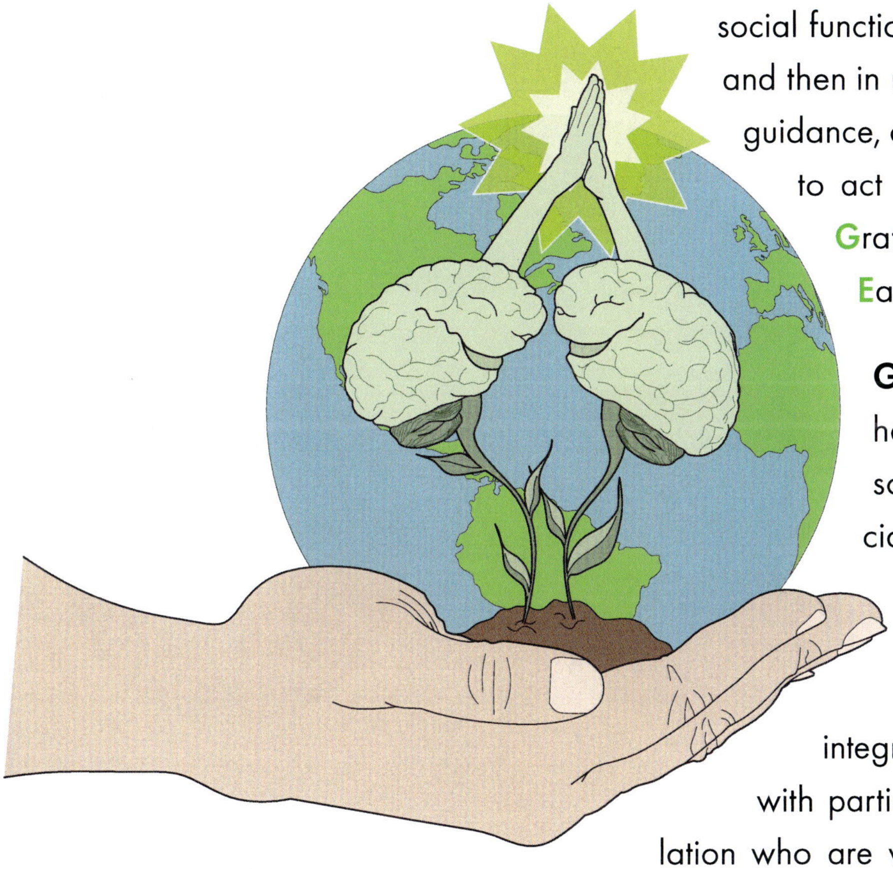

Growing G.R.E.E.N. InterActions has been developed to foster social analysis skills and prosocial behavior in individuals with emotional and pragmatic language challenges. However, the program's concepts and integrative activities also are effective with participants from the general population who are working to improve their social skills.

The target population for this program is students in third grade through middle school, but some lessons and approaches have been used successfully with younger students as well. Other lessons and strategies have proved useful with high school students and adults who can benefit from developing prosocial skills.

Thoughts, feelings, and behavior can be visualized as a triangle with each part affecting the others. Our thoughts influence how we perceive what happens around us, which in turn strongly influences our feelings about it. Our feelings then affect our behavior, which is how we act in the situation. The process continues in a loop, with our behavior reinforcing our thoughts, which continue to affect our feelings. If one part of the "triangle" is negative, every corner is influenced.

If our thoughts affect how we feel, and how we feel affects our behavior, we can benefit from cognitive–behavioral therapy. That approach allows us to see whether an individual's thoughts can be changed to result in more **positive** feelings. Such improved positivity results in more **positive** prosocial behavior. Given the **power** to change what we are thinking, we also can change how we feel and act. As participants are guided to be **thoughtful** instead of impulsive, they begin to consider alternative thoughts within structured situations, and in turn use those alternatives in less structured life interactions.

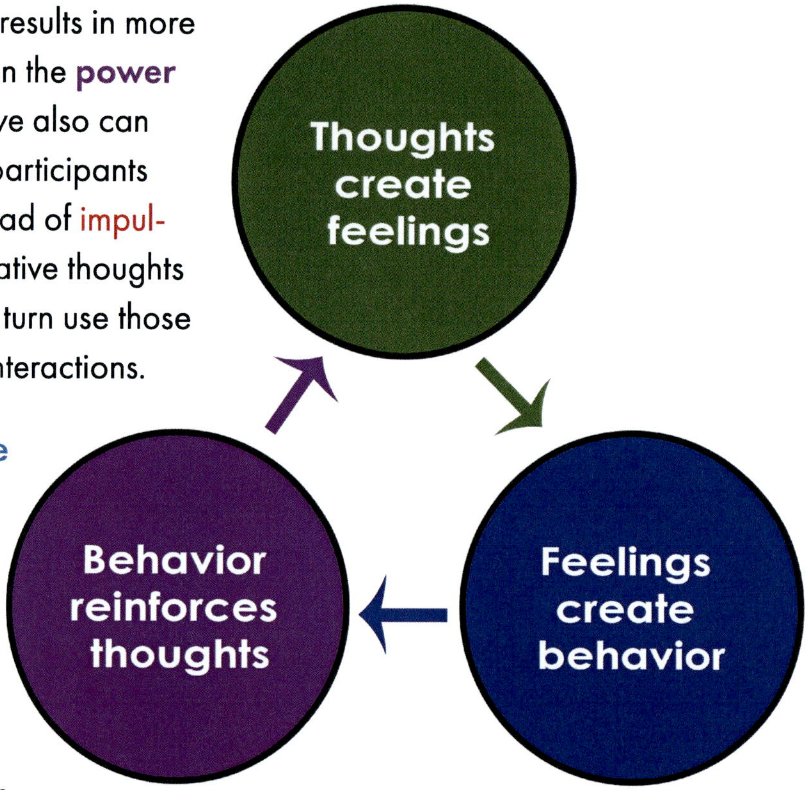

As they learn to **survey the scene** more carefully, paying attention to what and who is around them, they can include more of this information about others in their thoughts. This strategy best equips them to choose the most helpful, proactive thought. This positively affects their feelings and behavior simultaneously.

When working with me to present the **Growing G.R.E.E.N. InterActions** lessons and activities, Arielle, the school counselor, realized that this program helped guide **positive** changes in this thought–feeling–behavior triangle. She understood that, by explicitly presenting alternative prosocial thoughts ("**Guiding G.R.E.E.N. Thoughts**®") and related explicit scripts ("**G.R.E.E.N. Scenes**"), participants could think about and act out more prosocial behaviors. Through guided prosocial activities, participants associated prosocial thoughts with **positive** feelings. This resulted, at least in part, from positive reinforcement from the rest of the Team when G.R.E.E.N. action was exhibited. There appeared to be an increased likelihood that actual prosocial actions could be elicited using these methods. This prosocial G.R.E.E.N. behavior and its subsequent reinforcement strengthened the power of using **Guiding G.R.E.E.N. Thoughts**, with participants starting to think of them and use them on their own.

The more a participant reaches for and uses a prosocial **Guiding G.R.E.E.N. Thought**, the easier it becomes to substitute it for less reinforcing thoughts. For this to work, attention must be placed on reinforcing newer, positive behavior rather than negative. Some individuals have only learned to get attention by acting out in negative ways. Negative behavior is more commonly pointed out because it affects the forward movement of the scene and needs to be dealt with before the scene becomes even worse.

"Catch me being good" is sometimes more difficult to do because people are less likely to provide positive reinforcement when things are going well. To allow for the effectiveness of this reinforcement in developing positive feelings and ongoing productivity, deliberate effort is needed in order to stop to reinforce the actions of those acting well in a situation that is already going well. By focusing on positive rather than negative reinforcement, we create a better chance of making positive changes and reducing maladaptive, antisocial behavior.

The **Growing G.R.E.E.N. InterActions Social Literacy Program** is aligned with key concepts and advice provided in an excellent, classic anger management book used widely by psychologists and social workers, *When Anger Hurts*, by Matthew McKay, PhD, Peter D. Rogers, PhD, and Judith McKay, RN. It provides instruction and tools for individuals to notice, take charge of, and change maladaptive behaviors. Several key concepts in this classic treatment resource are aligned with those of the **Growing G.R.E.E.N. InterActions Program**:

1. ***Increasing personal responsibility for actions allows for improved behavior.***

   The **Growing G.R.E.E.N. InterActions Program** increases personal responsibility by increasing participants' awareness that they each have a powerful brain, with which they can make wise choices that can positively affect any Team they are on.

2. ***Strategies are needed for combating trigger thoughts.***

   A trigger thought is one that "triggers" a negative action. **Growing G.R.E.E.N. InterActions** guides participants to develop awareness of impulsive thoughts so they can deliberately substitute them with adaptive **Guiding G.R.E.E.N. Thoughts**®. This can occur when one takes the time to Think First before taking action. By Thinking First and using **Wise Action Tool** strategies such as the Civilized **Choice Checker**, participants choose **Guiding G.R.E.E.N. Thoughts** that lead to G.R.E.E.N. actions benefiting participants and their Teams.

3. ***Healthy self-talk is a strategy that works.***

   Guiding oneself to positive prosocial thinking such as **Guiding G.R.E.E.N. Thoughts** is a structured version of healthy self-talk. The **Growing G.R.E.E.N. InterActions Program** provides many opportunities for participants to engage in this useful self-guiding strategy.

4. ***Improved self-awareness and self-control can stop the escalation of maladaptive behaviors.***

   Although difficult to achieve, stopping the escalation of negative behaviors is critical for our life scenes to move **forward positively** so that we achieve **Personal** and **Team Goals**. This program presents structure and concepts that help participants learn to become more self-aware of positive versus negative behaviors. Increased self-awareness allows them to develop the self-control skills to act in more positive ways more often. Participants learn the responsibility and skill of reading the signals that tell them a calming break may be needed. Guides can provide cues to participants when a calming break is needed but no self-calming action has been initiated. Participants become more aware of when they should stop because they are acting antisocial and R.E.D. They learn how to "flip the switch" and "Brake to Take a (self-calming) Five Break." They learn why putting on their brakes is a better choice than continuing with negative action. Participants learn that accepting cues from others and from their own bodies is better than avoiding or neglecting these feedback cues. Accepting and using feedback can make the scene better for everyone. They learn that being as calm as possible allows one to make the best action choices. Therefore, the first step to having a G.R.E.E.N. InterAction is for each participant to get calm and stay calm, no matter how they perceive others acting at that moment. Self-guiding thoughts can be chosen and used most effectively when participants are calmest.

2 Setting the Stage for Growing G.R.E.E.N. InterActions®

2.1 Formal Baselines

Teachers and therapists should obtain formal baselines to determine areas of need. Surveys can be provided to the participant's teacher or parents to determine which behaviors and social language skills the participant may find difficult. These can become target areas for improvement. One or more of the following profiles are suggested:

A. **CELF-5 PRAGMATICS PROFILE**—subtest of the *Clinical Evaluation of Language Fundamentals®—Fifth Edition (CELF®-5)* by Elisabeth H. Wiig, PhD, Eleanor Semel, EdD and Wayne A. Secord, PhD, available through Pearson: www.pearsonclinical.com.

B. **CELF-5 METALINGUISTICS PROFILE**—subtest of *CELF–5 Metalinguistics*, by Elisabeth H. Wiig, PhD and Wayne A. Secord, PhD, available through Pearson: www.pearsonclinical.com.

A total score can be obtained as a baseline from either profile. Rankings for specific areas of difficulty, defined as 1 (never or almost never observed) and 2 (sometimes observed) are even more useful. These profiles can be completed again after 6 to 9 months to see whether progress has been made with targeted behaviors.

C. A completed **Assessment of Lagging Skills and Unsolved Problems (ALSUP)** also can be used as a baseline. This discussion guide from Ross Greene's "Lives in the Balance" program helps lead discussion among therapist, teacher, and parent to determine which lagging skills and unsolved problems to address (www.livesinthebalance.org).

D. This program's G.R.E.E.N. **Actions Evaluation** worksheet can be copied and filled out by participants and their teachers and parents. A total score can be obtained for each separate evaluation. This can act as the baseline for how G.R.E.E.N. each evaluator considers the participant. Comparing participants' views of their behavior with those of their teachers and parents can be useful. Participants commonly rate their functioning as higher than others rate it. When the evaluation chart is updated 6 to 9 months later, results often show increased similarity across different evaluators, as the participant has learned how to act G.R.E.E.N. and be a better self-assessor while learning.

2.2 Describing What It Means to Be G.R.E.E.N.

Explain what it means to be civilized and G.R.E.E.N. using the lessons in Section 1.2 of the ***Lesson Book***. Reinforce participant behavior by presenting participants with tokens on the **G.R.E.E.N. Token Tracker** found in the Interactive Toolbox. Initiate discussions about developing good character by taking steps to act G.R.E.E.N. in the scenes of our lives. Stress the importance of being a character with good character.

2.3 Songs Related to Lessons

Play the ***Songs for Guiding G.R.E.E.N. Thoughts*** album before, during, or after lessons so participants can hear the prosocial messages that relate to the program.

2.4 Lesson Logs

Guides should fill in the Lesson Log at the end of each lesson to summarize the main idea the participant was to learn. This should be done for whole group lessons as well. Review these lesson logs at the beginning of the next lesson so the guide can see how much participants remember and better connect one lesson to the next. The guide should keep a copy of this lesson log.

2.5 Self-Calming Lessons and Strategies

If participants need self-calming strategies in order to attend to **Growing G.R.E.E.N. InterActions** lessons, provide them with the strategies and songs found in Section 13 of the ***Lesson Book***. Guided breathing is presented with Song 5, "Brake to Take a Five Break."

2.6 Being on Teams, Team Rules, and Thinking First

Guides should present lessons about being on Teams and how Thinking First benefits the Team. Providing these lessons and **Wise Action Tools** helps participants realize they are on Teams with others and have the power to help their Teams achieve

Common Team Goals. Related lessons can be found in Section 4 of the ***Lesson Book***. Work together with the Team to establish rules that let it continue to move forward. Copy an appropriate Team Rules page, fill it out with the Team, and post it for everyone's reference. Begin to present lessons on how to Think First to make the best choices for positive consequences. Find related lessons in "Thinking First to Make Best Choices," which is Section 11 of the ***Lesson Book***.

2.7 Initial Lessons, Personal Goals, and Guiding G.R.E.E.N. Thoughts

Guides should choose initial lessons, Personal Goals, and **Guiding G.R.E.E.N. Thoughts** based on areas of need noted in evaluations. The decision about which concept to focus on first may be made using the baseline evaluations discussed earlier in this chapter. Present initial lessons related to the concept vocabulary and behavior that are most beneficial for participants to learn. Most participants also benefit from the lessons about reducing impulsivity and making choices for positive consequences included in Section 11.5 of the ***Lesson Book***. Participants may also benefit from initial lessons on **navigating** (Section 28) and **transformations** (Section 15).

After reviewing the lesson on realistic goal setting, conduct guided discussions to assist the participant in developing an initial Personal Goal "to be your best self in your Best Life." Help participants choose goals for targeted behaviors that should lead to positive differences in their interactions with others (see also the Personal Goals section). Help participants review their Personal Goal worksheets on a weekly basis to determine whether they have made progress toward their goal.

Provide participants with personally relevant **Guiding G.R.E.E.N. Thoughts** as visual aids as they make their best choices (see also the ***Lesson Book*** section "Getting Power from **Guiding G.R.E.E.N. Thoughts**").

2.8 Reinforcing Participant Actions

Guides should frequently reinforce participant actions by writing out, sharing, and tracking **G.R.E.E.N. Action Reports**. These reports show participants that you have noticed their successful attempts to act prosocial and G.R.E.E.N. in structured and unstructured situations. Describe the G.R.E.E.N. action and briefly tell how it positively affects the whole Team. Schedule a weekly time for the Team to share the G.R.E.E.N. action that was demonstrated by each Team member. This can be a time to celebrate the Team getting stronger and moving forward toward its goal. Give participants further credit for attaining these G.R.E.E.N. **Action Reports** by noting the prosocial action on Personal and Team G.R.E.E.N. **Action Trackers**.

2.9 Quick G.R.E.E.N. Scenes

Guides can check how well participants act G.R.E.E.N. by providing **Quick** G.R.E.E.N. **Scenes**. Several **Quick** G.R.E.E.N. **Scenes** can be used to obtain baseline performance with and without scripts. You may start with the Basic Skills G.R.E.E.N. **Scenes**.

2.10 Lessons About Acting Empathetically

Some important basic skills are taught in the ***Lesson Book*** sections on acting empathetic. Once participants display self-control and learn to be thoughtful instead of impulsive, they then can focus on becoming more aware of how others are feeling and what can be said to them in basic conversations. Participants can learn to infer what others are feeling and provide some basic relevant, appropriate things to say. Lessons about acting empathetically are found in Section 20 of the ***Lesson Book***. Participants can learn about being empathetic as they learn about being grateful and respectful, before developing the more complex skills needed to be easygoing.

2.11 Early Use of Priority Lessons

The ***Lesson Book*** is structured for use in the order written. However, presenting some priority lessons earlier may benefit certain participants.

Please review the Table of Contents to familiarize yourself with the concepts, interactive lessons, and G.R.E.E.N. **Scenes** in choosing what to present to your Team to help it grow more G.R.E.E.N.

3 Components of the Growing G.R.E.E.N. InterActions Program®

3.1 *InterActive Lesson Book*

Lessons and exercises provide participants with the foundational concepts and social literacy needed to develop social Team awareness and Common Team Goals. Explicit lessons on acting G.R.E.E.N. are paired with **Guiding** G.R.E.E.N. **Thoughts**® that participants can use when taking action in motivating, scripted G.R.E.E.N. **Scenes**.

3.2 *Guide's Guide* Instructor's Manual

The Guide's Guide is an instruction manual for becoming an effective guide of pro-social InterActions. It provides an explanation of the critical concepts and strategies integral to the program. It explains the instructional tools and tracking sheets that the guide can use to implement the program. This includes **Wise Action Tools**, which are visual strategies and worksheets that can be referred to and utilized by participants in structured lessons and real-life situations.

3.3 InterActive Toolbox

The Toolbox includes a variety of hands-on items used to focus, direct, and motivate program participants. The Toolbox's engaging items, visual aids, and positive reinforcement tools dramatically improve results and make the program more enjoyable and effective:

- G.R.E.E.N. **Scene Clapboard** for participants to act out scenes as if on a movie set. This tool motivates participant performances and additional "takes" of G.R.E.E.N. **Scenes** for further improvement by signaling a "Take 2." Conversations can also be "redone" so that they include critical elements and suggested scripts.

- G.R.E.E.N. **Token Trackers** pad and G.R.E.E.N. **Tokens** bag, for reinforcing target behaviors during lessons.

- G.R.E.E.N. **Action Report Cards** for guides to note the specific G.R.E.E.N. behaviors that they observe. The participant can review the feedback and share it with others. Participants also can give cards to peers to credit their G.R.E.E.N. behavior.
- **Guiding** G.R.E.E.N. **Thoughts Fidget Brain** that can be used as both a self-calming strategy and a self-focusing tool.
- **Guiding** G.R.E.E.N. **Thoughts affirmation cards** (36, preprinted) encourage thinking that assists participants in making prosocial choices. Also included is a sticky-pad of blank **Guiding** G.R.E.E.N. **Thoughts** to allow guides and participants to write personally relevant, **powerful** affirmations that can be kept and reviewed anywhere.
- A **program-specific album** comprising positive songs that encourage and reinforce team-centered social interactions.

4 Key Concepts of Growing G.R.E.E.N. InterActions®

Before engaging participants in learning to act prosocially, guides should become familiar with several key concepts integral to **Growing G.R.E.E.N. InterActions**.

4.1 Act Civilized and G.R.E.E.N. and Avoid Acting R.E.D.—G.R.E.E.N. Actions Can Help Our Civilization Move Forward

Of course, knowing what it means to act G.R.E.E.N. is important, as it allows you to effectively teach and model this kind of behavior to those you are guiding. G.R.E.E.N. is an acronym that stands for ways to act prosocially (Grateful, Respectful, Empathetic, Easygoing and Navigating). The program provides lessons teaching how to act in these ways. Participants also are provided situations to analyze in order to determine whether G.R.E.E.N. choices have been made by the characters. Participants are then guided to act G.R.E.E.N. in real-life scenes through the reinforcement tools integral to the program. One is the G.R.E.E.N. **Token Tracker** (Figure 1), which the guide can begin to use during the first lesson to tangibly reinforce cooperative, G.R.E.E.N. behavior:

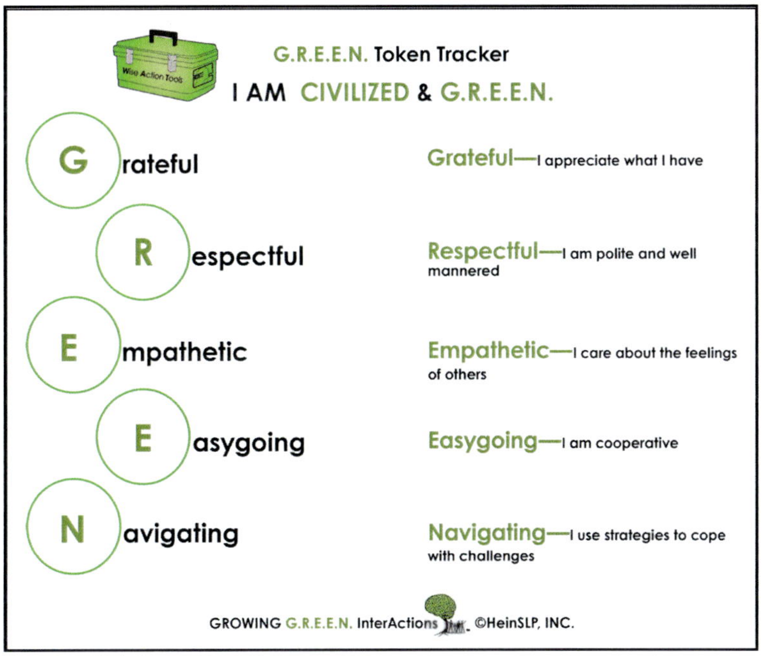

Figure 1. G.R.E.E.N. Token Tracker

Participants will find G.R.E.E.N. actions contrasted with the R.E.D. behavior we want to avoid. Its letters stand for **R**ude, **E**gocentric, and **D**isruptive (Figure 2). Participants can ask themselves or be asked by others what action choices they are making:

G.R.E.E.N. Behavior	R.E.D. Behavior
Grateful Respectful Empathetic Easygoing Navigating	Rude Egocentric Disruptive

Figure 2. G.R.E.E.N. and R.E.D. behaviors defined

It is important to present the idea that we are not only contrasting G.R.E.E.N. and R.E.D. choices in our lives, but also choosing among G.R.E.E.N. and G.R.E.E.N.-er actions.

A section of the program highlights our civilization's dependence on living and working together in a cooperative, civil way. The first song on the album ***Songs for Guiding G.R.E.E.N. Thoughts***, "Keep the Civil in Civilization," carries this message.

This program includes scenarios in which participants analyze scenes with R.E.D. behavior and "change the scene to make it G.R.E.E.N." They help the characters make better choices in their words and actions. **Quick G.R.E.E.N. Scenes** guide participants to follow short prosocial scripts, whereas longer **G.R.E.E.N. Scenes** provide explicit scripts for what participants can say to be prosocial in more complex situations. It is critical that participants only act out **G.R.E.E.N. Scenes**, avoiding R.E.D. ones. Some participants ask whether they may act out R.E.D. Scenes, but they are told that the behaviors in R.E.D. Scenes do not need to be rehearsed! R.E.D. behavior is not the target we want to encourage!

4.2 Make Life Better by Using Wise Action Tools

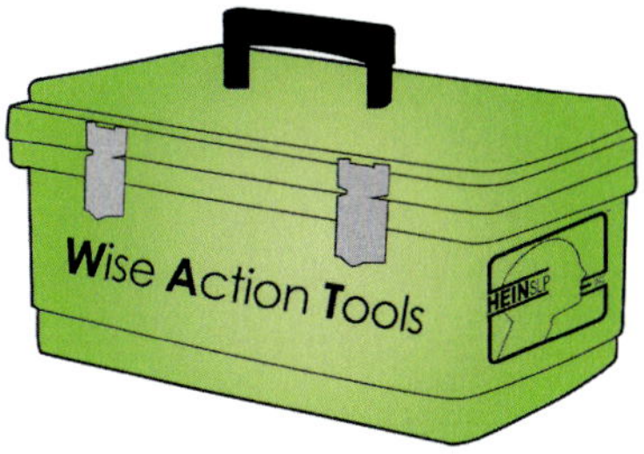

Wise Action Tools are visual strategies, integral to this program, that assist participants in analyzing social information and acting in systematic ways. Participants are guided to use **Wise Action Tools** when engaged in lessons and structured activities, but also are encouraged to use these tools in real-life social interactions.

Wise Action Tools and behavioral reinforcements guide participants to develop specific skills:

- increasing awareness of being on Teams
- setting goals with Teams
- establishing Team rules
- evaluating and tracking G.R.E.E.N. action
- picturing your **Best Life**
- setting and tracking progress on **Personal Goals**
- Thinking First by using affirmations called **Guiding G.R.E.E.N. Thoughts®** to guide the best action choices
- using choice checkers to systematically determine which of two actions to choose
- thoroughly analyzing and **surveying** social scenes with a structured organizer
- using self-calming strategies
- engaging in personal **transformations**
- developing appreciation for what one has
- answering questions without delay
- being on topic
- engaging in conversation on nonpreferred topics
- using appropriate tone of voice and vocal volume
- being aware of one's audience when choosing topics
- taking action to connect consistently with others
- choosing to show **positive** feelings and **positive** action
- engaging in **cooperative conversations**
- accepting constructive feedback
- making **compromises**
- increasing awareness of when one should ask for help

4.3 Survey the Scene before Choosing What Is Best to Do or Say

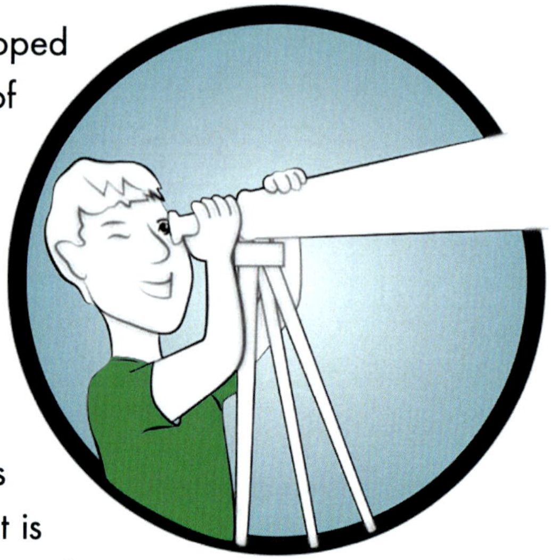

Speech-language pathologist Herb Hein developed this program to increase the social literacy of his students and clients. His program focuses heavily on guiding participants to effectively process social information—paying attention to what they are seeing, hearing, or reading—in order to better understand social situations. This program stresses the active **surveying** of information by participants to find details and clues from which they can best guess what is happening in the social scenes presented to them. The guide assists in interpreting these social clues and details, and participant responses and interactions can be directed toward increasingly on-target and prosocial behavior.

To develop analysis skills, program participants are guided to "**survey the scene**" (Figure 3).

They are asked to analyze character actions and words in sentences, stories, and scenarios to determine whether they are being **helpful** and **prosocial** (**G.R.E.E.N.**) or hurtful and antisocial (R.E.D.). Participants develop social literacy through lessons that help them perceive and analyze the salient social details in each scene.

Participants are subsequently guided to become better at **surveying** and analyzing real-life scenes so they can best choose how to act with the people in their lives.

This program provides many opportunities for participants to analyze situations so they become more empathetic and can accurately assess how someone might be feeling. They are then guided to determine the best thing to do or say. The "**Survey the Scene to Infer How Others Are Feeling**" section of the ***Lesson Book*** provides scripts to help participants know what to say to match a person's feelings. In the subsequent section, participants are challenged by scenarios where they must determine for themselves the best thing to say to act empathetic and supportive.

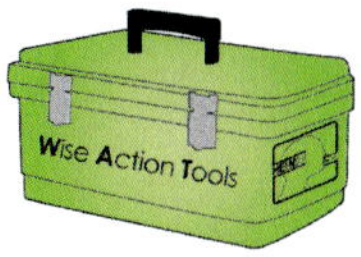

SURVEYING THE SCENE BEFORE TAKING ACTION

Directions: As you read each G.R.E.E.N. Scene, find clues to help you answer the following questions. This will help you know how to act in the scene.

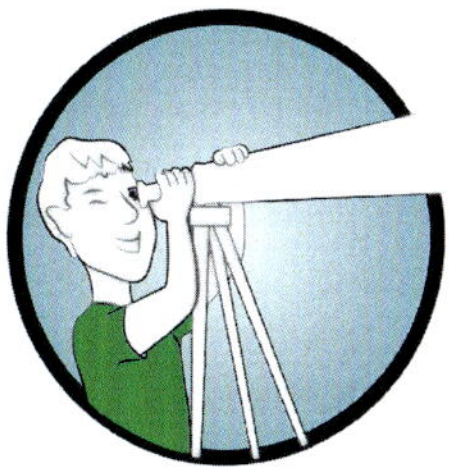

1. The name of this G.R.E.E.N. Scene is ______________________________

2. What is the setting (where is this scene happening)? ______________________________

____

3. Who are the characters (who is in this scene)? ______________________________

____

4. What kind of Team is in this scene? Home Team School Team Friendship Team

5. What does each character in this scene want or need? ______________________________

____

____

6. What do you think is the Common Team Goal in this scene? ______________________________

____

7. What would be a positive consequence of everyone in the scene doing their best to act G.R.E.E.N.?

____

Growing G.R.E.E.N. InterActions® HeinSLP, Inc. www.heinslpinc.com

Figure 3. Surveying the Scene worksheet

4.4 Be Team-Oriented!

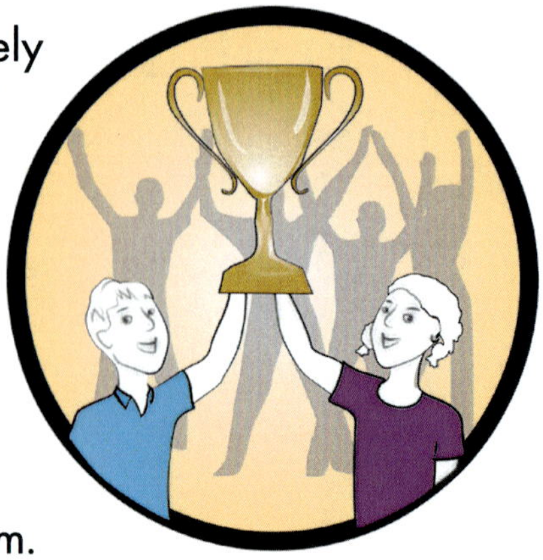

A critical concept of this program is that we are more likely to use our best actions when we consider ourselves part of various Teams in our lives. We do not live in our modern society on our own. For society to move **forward**, we must think beyond our individual needs, wants, and feelings to realize that the people in our life scenes are as important as we are. Participants may have emotional or neurological challenges that make it difficult for them to perceive that other people are on the same Team. Despite these challenges, improving their awareness, understanding, and skills in Team-connecting is still possible.

This program provides vocabulary, scenarios, scripts, and integrative activities to increase participant awareness of being on a Team with other people in scripted and "real-life" scenes. These include Class, Home, and Friendship Teams as well as community groups with whom the participant interacts. **Growing G.R.E.E.N. InterActions** provides guided practice to help the participant experience how Team-focused, prosocial action looks, sounds, and feels.

Participants are asked to write down the types of Teams and the people on them. Naming Teams and their members helps participants realize that they are not alone in these settings and situations. Being on Teams guides participants to make mutually beneficial choices instead of only individual ones. Participants are guided to become aware of the **Common Team Goals** so their choices will support the Team's goals. The material in the program continually supports the participant in becoming more Team-centric. Participants begin to consider, "Will this action help the Team move **forward** toward reaching its goals?"

4.5 Using Common Team Goals to Guide Action Choices

Naming the **Common Team Goal** allows everyone to understand it and work toward meeting it. This unified effort to achieve a goal is quite **powerful**. But even more **powerful** is printing it out and posting it where it can be seen regularly by everyone on the Team. The **Common Team Goal** for the classroom, home, and other important settings should be spelled out and posted in a visible location so Team members can refer to it often.

The concept of all members acting G.R.E.E.N. for the Team can be integrated into all home and school activities. This helps Team members perceive positive changes in the environment when the Team works together to meet the Common Team Goal (Figure 4).

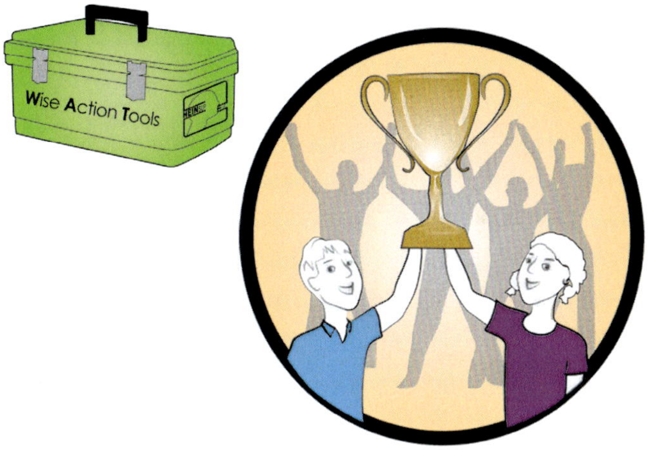

OUR TEAM NAME ______________________________

OUR COMMON TEAM GOALS

____

____

____

____

____

____

Growing G.R.E.E.N. InterActions® HeinSLP, Inc. www.heinslpinc.com

Figure 4. Common Team Goals worksheet

4.6 Connecting with Your Team through G.R.E.E.N. Actions and by Developing Consistently Prosocial Behavior

Students are guided to choose G.R.E.E.N. behavior, and positive reinforcement is given for making G.R.E.E.N. choices and acting G.R.E.E.N. The program provides **Quick G.R.E.E.N. Scenes** so guides can assess how well participants act G.R.E.E.N., on their own or with scripts modeling what to say and how to say it. Participants receive feedback so they know how they have performed.

It should be clearly communicated to participants that when they act G.R.E.E.N., they help their Team meet its goal. The positive consequences of acting G.R.E.E.N. are highlighted throughout the program and should be discussed often. As participants are guided to act prosocially, they learn to perceive how their actions positively affect their Home, Class, and Friendship Teams.

Program participants strengthen their abilities to navigate challenges and perceive how others are feeling. They are guided to develop skills for taking steps to positively connect with other Team members. You may guide this process through visual techniques such as the **Connection Direction Tracker**. Structured activities such as **Quick G.R.E.E.N. Scenes** challenge participants to move a token in Team-connecting directions four times in a row when asked for a verbal response. They are encouraged to act consistently G.R.E.E.N. with their words, their tone, and other behaviors considered positive, prosocial, and Team-connecting. The **Connection Direction Tracker** is thus a means to shape participant behavior and consistency for at least four "takes." They can have as many opportunities as needed until their responses become consistent and automatic.

The **Connection Direction Tracker** visual strategy (Figure 5) helps guide and strengthen the concept of consistent G.R.E.E.N. actions and can be used as participants develop other respectful and easygoing skills:

- using a polite, respectful tone
- following Team rules
- taking turns to share information
- listening when the other person is talking
- asking questions about the other person's topic

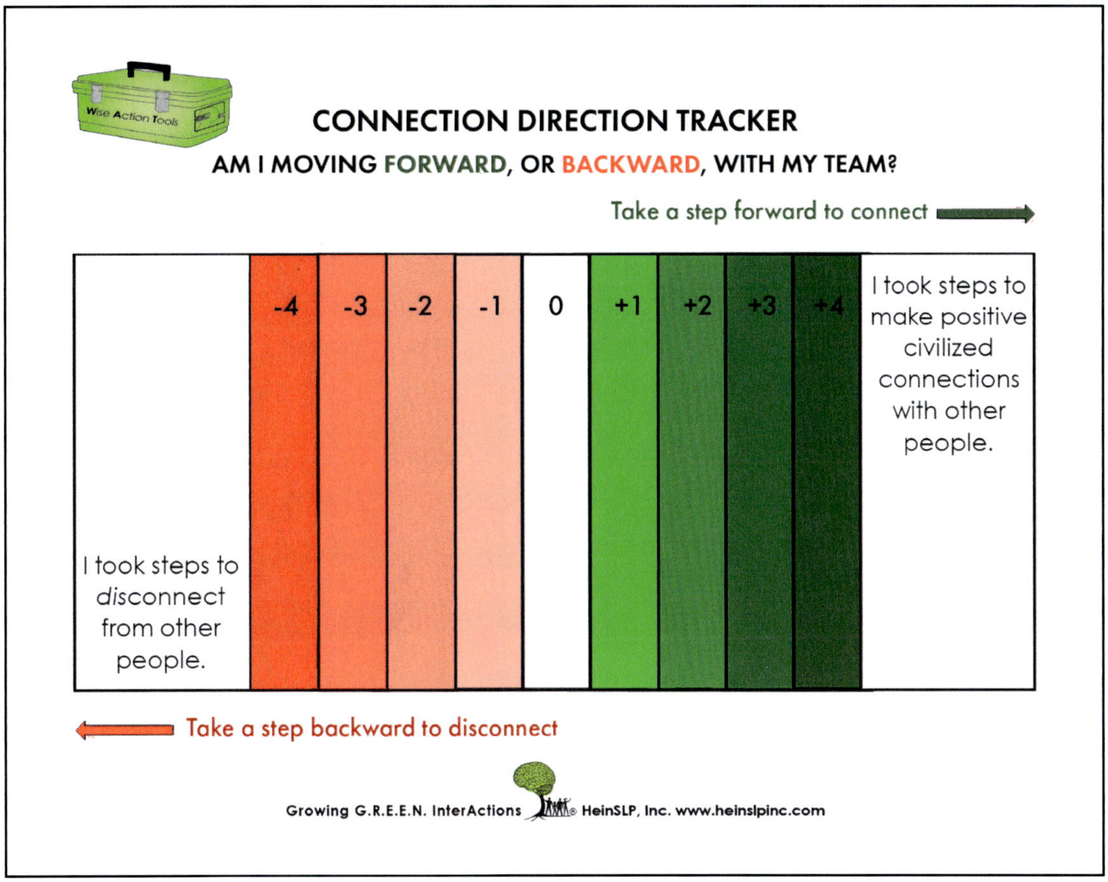

Figure 5. Connection Direction Tracker

4.7 Honestly Evaluating Behavior

This program includes a G.R.E.E.N. **Actions Evaluation Chart** for the participant and guide to complete. This helps establish a baseline of performance to determine areas for G.R.E.E.N. growth.

Initially participants may find it difficult to engage in honest self-assessment. But engaging in the self-assessment process leads participants to think more frequently about their interactions with other Team members. As G.R.E.E.N. language is provided and target behavior is introduced in lessons and activities, participants begin to see whether they are truly exhibiting the targeted behavior.

More honest self-assessment can be achieved by modeling the target behavior and providing opportunities for participants to engage in it. In this way, they discover what it feels like to act G.R.E.E.N. and whether they are choosing to act that way. Participants also feel the positive consequences of making G.R.E.E.N. action choices (Figure 6).

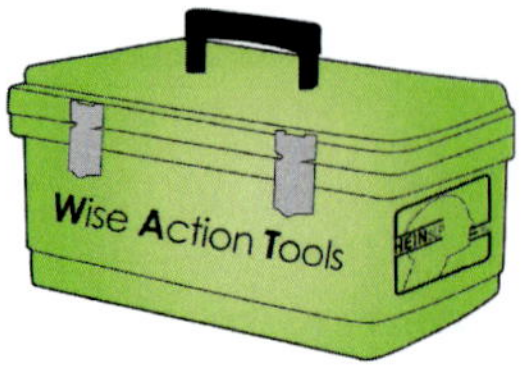

G.R.E.E.N. ACTIONS EVALUATION CHART

Team Member: ______________________________ Today's Date ____________________

Evaluation by:

- ☐ Self
- ☐ Teacher
- ☐ Parent
- ☐ Peer
- ☐ Other ________________

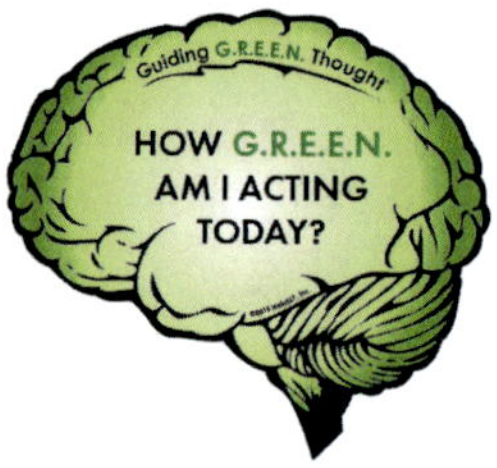

HONESTLY EVALUATE ACTIONS BY CHECKING THE BOX THAT IS TRUE TODAY

	NEVER 0	A LITTLE BIT 1	HALF THE TIME 2	MOST OF THE TIME 3	ALL THE TIME 4	TOTAL
GRATEFUL- I let people know that I appreciate what I have.						
RESPECTFUL- I am respectful of the people and things in every situation. I use a tone of voice that is positive and polite.						
EMPATHETIC- I show that I am considerate of the feelings of my friends, classmates, and family.						
EASYGOING- I am open-minded and cooperate with people to meet Team goals.						
NAVIGATING- I am flexible when I manage challenges because I stay calm and make wise choices.						
I take responsibility for my actions and accept consequences.						
				GRAND TOTAL		

Growing G.R.E.E.N. InterActions® HeinSLP, Inc. www.heinslpinc.com

Figure 6. G.R.E.E.N. Actions Evaluation Chart

4.8 Learn the Reasons for Rules So They Are Easier to Follow

The **Growing G.R.E.E.N. InterActions Program** includes lessons for determining each Team's rules so that Team members can navigate with one another and more easily act easygoing. It also highlights that participants are more likely to follow rules if they know why the rules exist and how they benefit the forward movement of the Team. Time should be taken to have Teams work together to establish mutually beneficial rules and to have everyone understand how those rules benefit the Team. The rules can then be posted for easy reference. **Wise Action Tool** sheets (Figure 7) allow rules to be spelled out for Home, Classroom, and Friendship Teams.

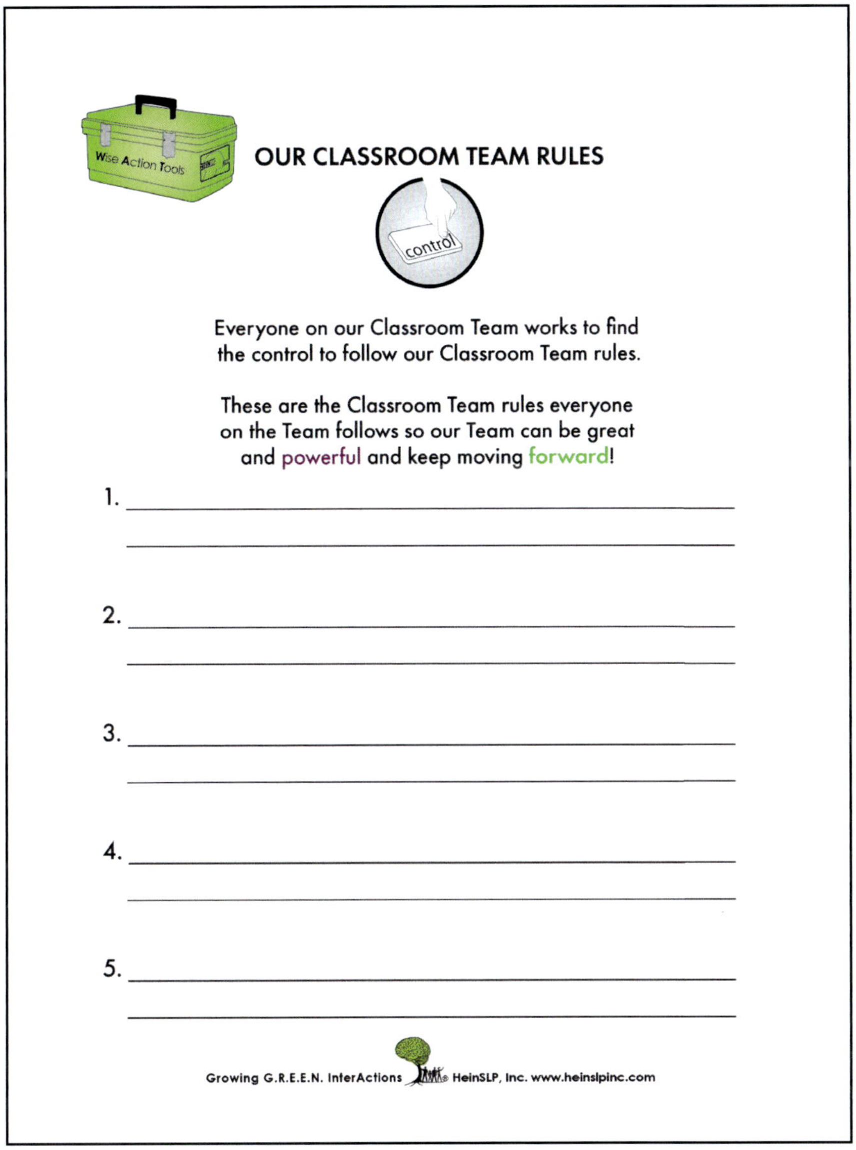
Wise Action Tools

OUR CLASSROOM TEAM RULES

control

Everyone on our Classroom Team works to find the control to follow our Classroom Team rules.

These are the Classroom Team rules everyone on the Team follows so our Team can be great and powerful and keep moving forward!

1. ______

2. ______

3. ______

4. ______

5. ______

Growing G.R.E.E.N. InterActions HeinSLP, Inc. www.heinslpinc.com

Figure 7. Classroom Team Rules worksheet

4.9 Benefiting from the Feedback of Others

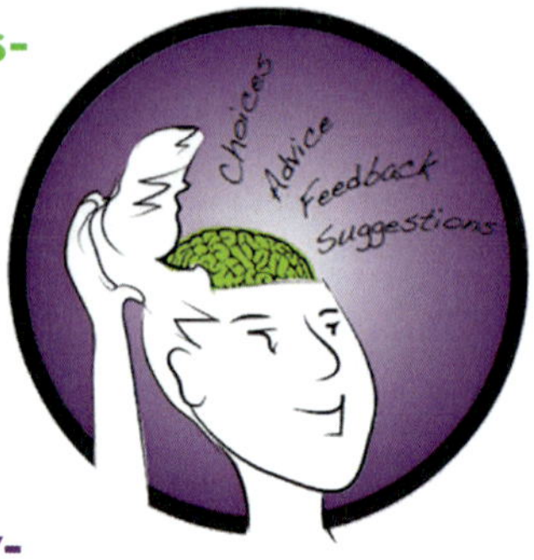

This program encourages participants to give one another positive feedback as often as possible. The more often positive feedback is given, the more the positive behavior is reinforced. One way Team members can support one another is by noticing the G.R.E.E.N. actions of others and reinforcing them with G.R.E.E.N. **Action Reports** (Figure 8). Regularly reviewing these positive behavior notes as a Team is powerful. G.R.E.E.N. **Action Reports** can be kept in a special box or other location to be pulled out and shared by the Team on a weekly basis.

G.R.E.E.N. ACTION REPORT

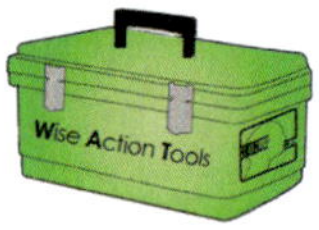

Date: ____________ Situation: ____________

____

Who acted G.R.E.E.N.? ______________________________

Circle the behavior(s) shown:

Grateful **R**espectful **E**mpathetic **E**asygoing **N**avigating

What was the G.R.E.E.N. action? ______________________________

____

____

GROWING G.R.E.E.N. InterActions® ©HeinSLP, INC.

Figure 8. G.R.E.E.N. Action Report

Negative feedback, when necessary, can be presented as constructive feedback, including the suggested positive change that will benefit the Team. This means the guide self-monitors how feedback is presented so that a positive behavioral choice is suggested. "It would be better for the Team right now if you took a break. After the break, we can discuss what might be a better choice for this situation." If feedback is given in this manner, participants find it easier to listen and respond in a favorable way. It guides flexible thinking as Team-benefiting action is presented as a choice to guide the participant to switch away from negative action.

4.10 Establish Realistic, Measurable Personal Goals and Strive to Meet Them

The importance of having Personal and Common Team Goals is explained in the first few sections of the ***Lesson Book***. Program worksheets can be used to establish Personal Goals (Figure 9).

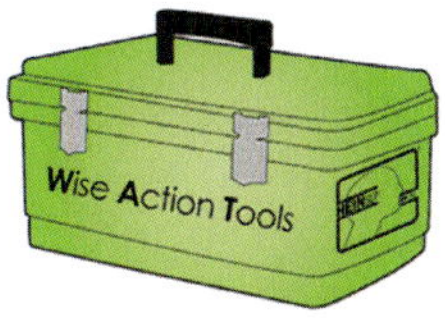

MY PERSONAL GOAL WORKSHEET

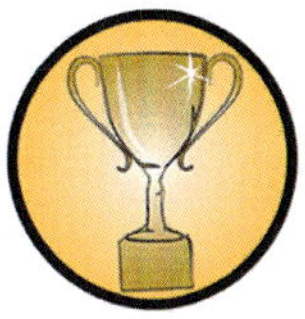

Today's Date: ____________________

Goal area: ____

My useful, realistic goal for the next week/month is: ________________

____

A. Baseline: Circle how often I do it today.

Never sometimes half of the time most of the time almost always

0 5 10 15 20 25 30 35 40 45 **50** 55 60 65 70 75 80 85 90 95 **100**

B. My realistic goal for the next week/month is to do this ______________ (how often?)

Never sometimes half of the time most of the time almost always

My Goal : How often will I be able to do the action written in my goal
(circle how far you can *realistically* move to the right):

0 5 10 15 20 25 30 35 40 45 **50** 55 60 65 70 75 80 85 90 95 **100**

Checking in: I am checking how I am doing on this date: ______________

How am I doing? ____

What am I doing well? ____

What can help me do better? ______________________________________

Growing G.R.E.E.N. InterActions® HeinSLP, Inc. www.heinslpinc.com

Figure 9. Personal Goal worksheet

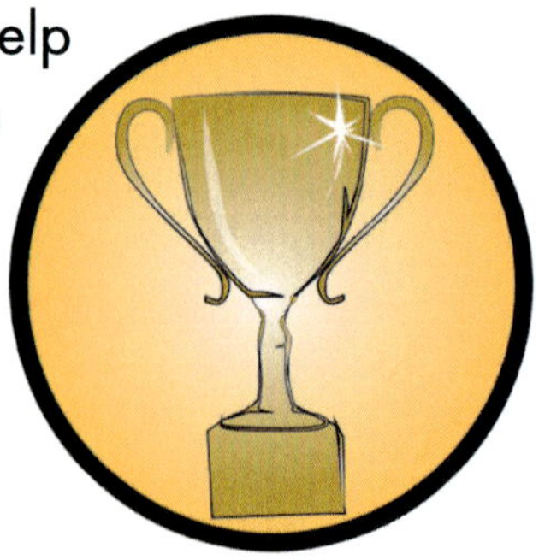

Teachers and therapists write goals to determine how to help their students and clients reach their social goals. Then the guide can encourage the participant to select that behavior as a **Personal Goal**, because in most cases it would benefit both the participant and the Team. Both the guide and the participant can then track how often the participant displays the related targeted action.

Participants can use the **Personal Goal** worksheet to establish realistic goals that can be achieved each month. It should include a baseline showing how often the behavior is exhibited initially, and what percentage of time the behavior is expected to be shown after a month (the target goal). Having specific goals for specific behaviors allows participants and guides to determine measurable improvement within a target area (Figure 10).

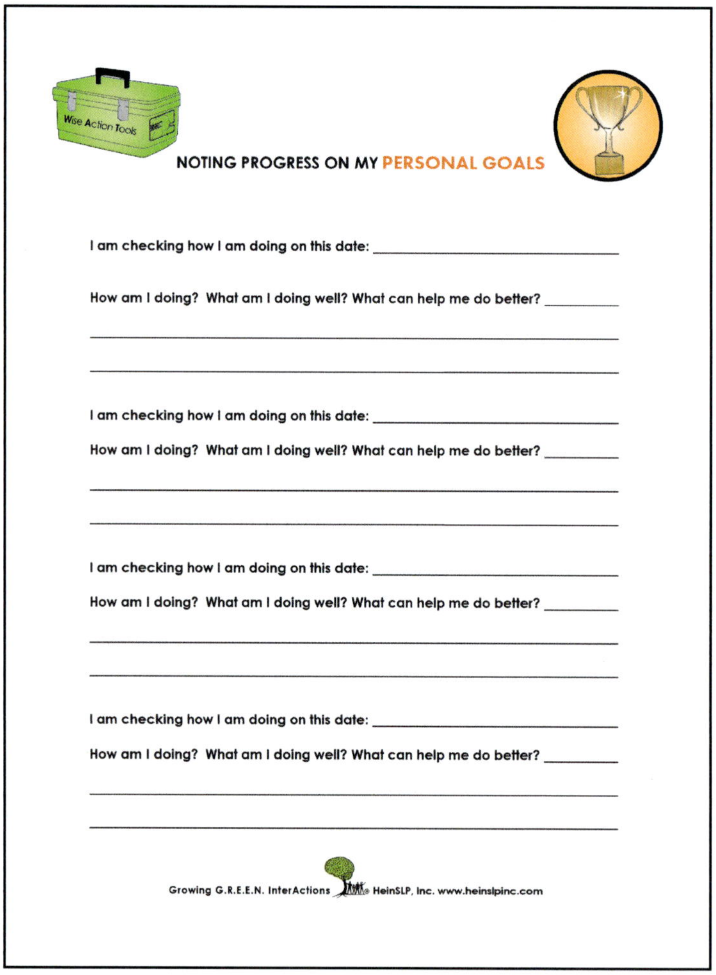

Wise Action Tools

NOTING PROGRESS ON MY PERSONAL GOALS

I am checking how I am doing on this date: ____________________

How am I doing? What am I doing well? What can help me do better? ________

____

____

I am checking how I am doing on this date: ____________________

How am I doing? What am I doing well? What can help me do better? ________

____

____

I am checking how I am doing on this date: ____________________

How am I doing? What am I doing well? What can help me do better? ________

____

____

I am checking how I am doing on this date: ____________________

How am I doing? What am I doing well? What can help me do better? ________

____

____

Growing G.R.E.E.N. InterActions HeinSLP, Inc. www.heinslpinc.com

Figure 10. Personal Goals Progress worksheet

4.11 Reach Up for Guiding G.R.E.E.N. Thoughts® to Take Powerful Steps Forward

A unique feature of this program is the inclusion of the explicit, manipulative affirmations called **Guiding G.R.E.E.N. Thoughts**. These brain-shaped, **positive** statements encourage participants to Think First and choose one guiding affirmation to help them make prosocial choices when interacting with others. Through the program's activities, the participant begins to perceive **Guiding G.R.E.E.N. Thoughts** can help the Team move **forward** rather than backward. When the Team moves **forward**, everyone can benefit. The participant is guided to see the **power** of using a thought to take action that makes a scene better.

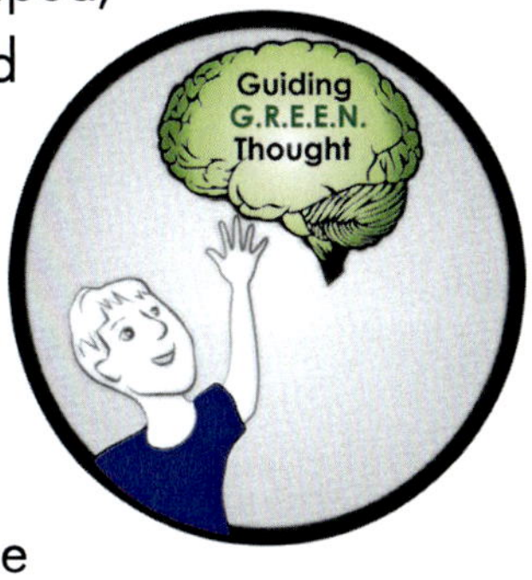

Guiding G.R.E.E.N. Thoughts, presented throughout the program, communicate many ideas that help us act in a cooperative, respectful, and mature way so we can be productive, prosocial citizens. They also guide us to use strategies to successfully navigate life's challenges. Many **Guiding G.R.E.E.N. Thoughts** have a related **G.R.E.E.N.** Scene to be acted out. These scenes can be taught in an explicit hands-on manner, allowing participants to analyze the affirmation's helpfulness and how the situation and people involved benefited from the targeted **Guiding G.R.E.E.N. Thought** (Figure 11 is a general example).

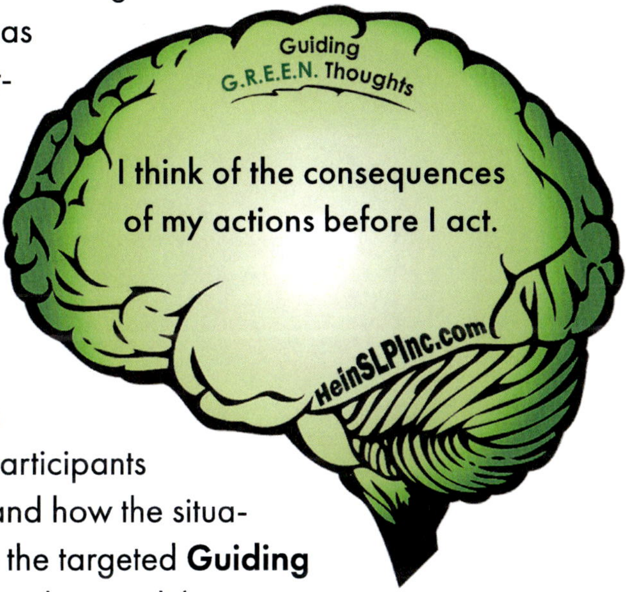

Figure 11. A Guiding G.R.E.E.N. Thought

4.12 Think First to Make the Best Choices

Prior to being introduced to this program, participants often do not understand or believe they can make good choices. They are ruled by their impulsive thoughts. A more optimistic and proactive view is that all human beings are capable of Thinking First before acting. This concept is presented early in the program. Participants are encouraged to turn on their human brain **power** and be open to the possibility that useful thoughts are available to help them make the best choices.

A powerful way to have participants begin to Think First in the moment is to guide them to think about four things before taking action: (1) Who is on the Team with me right now? (2) What is our **Common Team Goal**? (3) What do I want to accomplish right now—what is my **Personal Goal** for this moment? and (4) What **Guiding G.R.E.E.N. Thought** can help me meet my goal right now? By practicing the deliberate thinking needed to fill out this **Ready, Set, Goal!** worksheet, participants learn to be less impulsive, more goal directed, more capable of using guiding thoughts to be successful in subsequent follow-through, and better able to evaluate their own actions (Figure 12).

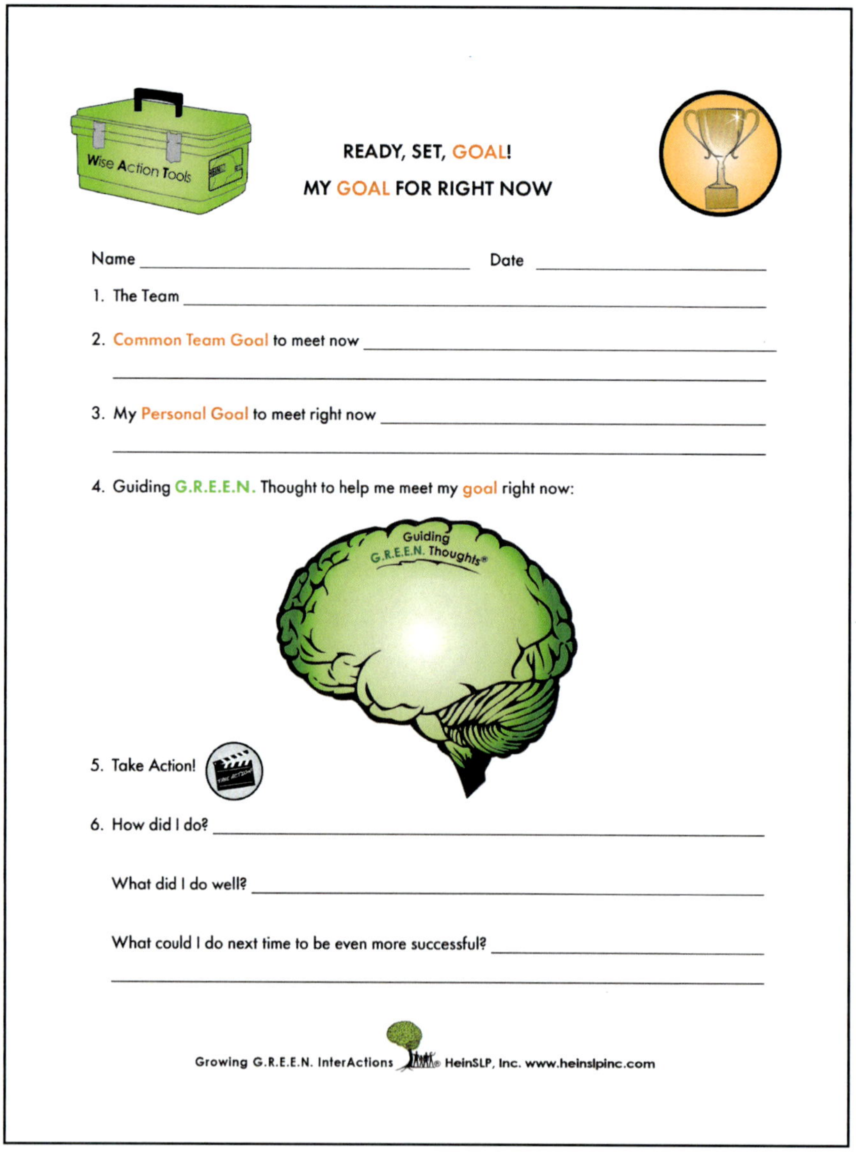

Figure 12. Ready, Set, Goal! planning worksheet

4.13 Get Calm and Stay Calm in Order to Think First

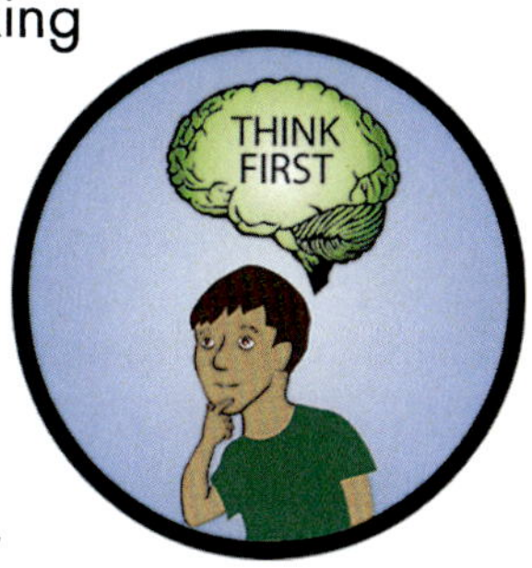

This program encourages participants to calm down before taking action so that their actions will be better for the Team. When our brain is in an agitated, excited state, we are less likely to make wise choices. In this state, our words and actions are more likely to be driven by our impulses. They are less likely to be put through our self-monitoring filter that asks, "How will this affect the others I am with?" As a guide, it is your responsibility to advise participants to delay choosing words or actions until they have time to allow their brains to return to a more calm, thoughtful state.

The program includes lessons that can be used to explain how humans can self-regulate. You can guide participants to see a "red light" in their brains telling them to "step on the brake," stop, and give themselves time to Think First. Guiding participants toward good action choices becomes much easier once they have learned this important skill. This program lets you guide participants to engage in visualization or the "Brake to Take a Five Break" controlled breathing strategy with musical cues on the album. Then, after getting calm, they can return to choosing the best thoughts that would lead to the best actions. Instead of thinking or saying, "I am so upset, I can't think!" your participant can think or say, "I will give myself a break so I can calm down. Then I can think of what to do next."

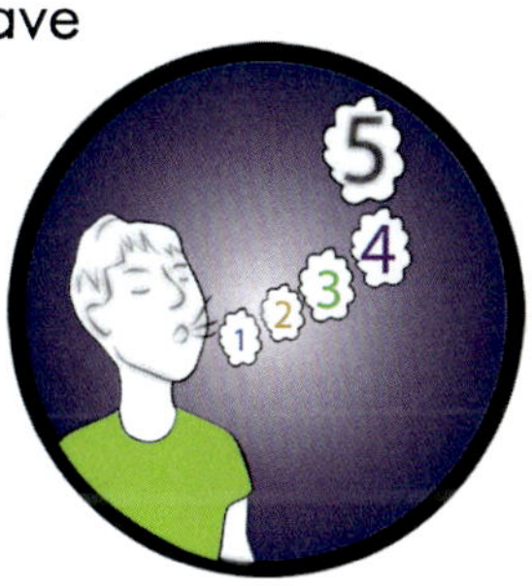

4.14 Step-by-Step Methods for Making the Best Choices

Depending on how well participants understand and display prosocial actions, some will need to learn the prerequisite concepts and behaviors for being G.R.E.E.N. presented in the first sections of the ***Lesson Book***.

Participants are guided to ask themselves:

- Is this action safe?
- Is this logical?
- Is this action good for everyone involved?

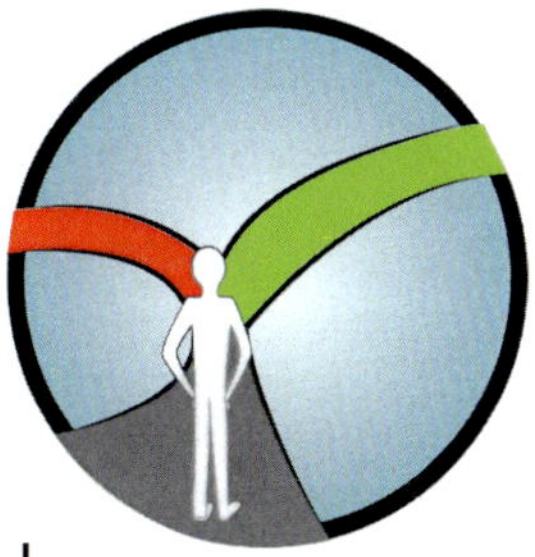

In contrast to the idea that some young people cannot understand these concepts because they are too abstract or complex, when guides explicitly present the vocabulary, it has been found that this population can understand it, especially when given concrete examples and contrasting ideas.

The program introduces specific lessons about what it means to act in a safe, logical, and good way for everyone. It explicitly provides examples of **positive** versus negative behavior and provides scripts to help participants perceive the consequences of those action choices. Comprehension of these cause-and-effect relationships of different action choices provides the foundation for participants to make their best life choices.

As social scenarios are discussed, participants are asked to think about whether characters are acting in the best, **positive** way to make the situation better. A **Civilized Choice Checker** (Figure 13) is presented when a character in a scene is making choices that would be considered R.E.D., and then has the chance to rewind or replay the scene to act more G.R.E.E.N. Participants judge whether each choice meets the criteria of being safe, logical, and good for everyone. Participants add up the **positive** check marks to see which choice wins. Participants are encouraged to use this **Civilized Choice Checker** whenever they must judge and choose among two or more actions.

4.15 Making Powerful Transformations

Participants learn to use **Guiding G.R.E.E.N. Thoughts** as they see characters in presented scenarios making **transformations** in their thoughts and actions. After guides have helped participants analyze these stories, participants are guided and encouraged to make **powerful transformations**, generating self-guiding thoughts and **transformative** movement toward improvement in their own stories. They can be guided to use the

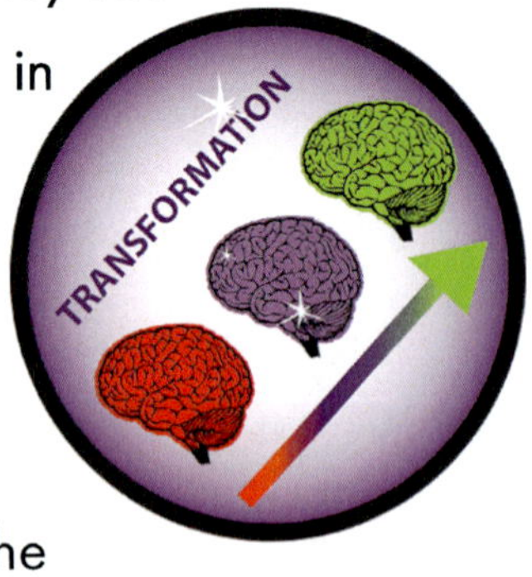

Thought Transformation Scene Changer (Figure 14) for analyzing **transformations** presented in the program's scenarios, and then be guided to use it to make **powerful transformations** in their own lives with their Teams.

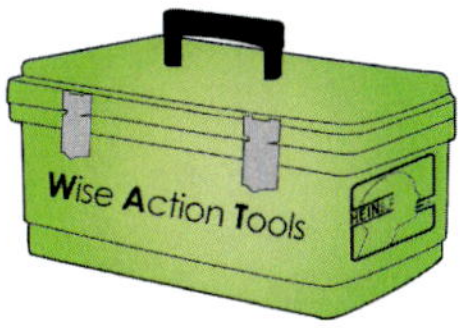

CIVILIZED CHOICE CHECKER

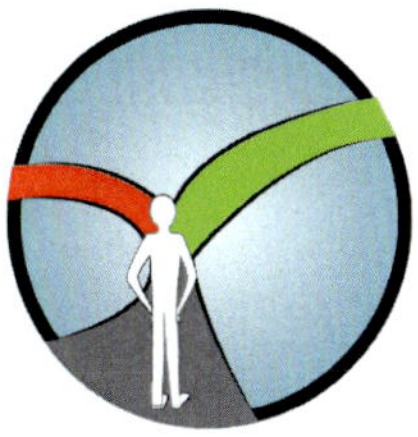

When I **survey this scene**, I think this is happening:

____

This is one way to act **(Choice A)**: ______________________________________

____

This is another way to act **(Choice B)**: ____________________________________

____

	Write "+" for yes and "-" for **no**	
	Action Choice A	Action Choice B
1. This is a logical choice. Things will get better instead of worse.		
2. This is a safe choice. People will *not* get hurt. Things will *not* get broken.		
3. This choice is good for everyone. Things will be better for *everyone* in the scene.		
4. This choice uses good self-control to meet the goals.		
Total score: Add up the + signs to see which choice is the best. Which choice wins?		

Figure 13. Civilized Choice Checker worksheet

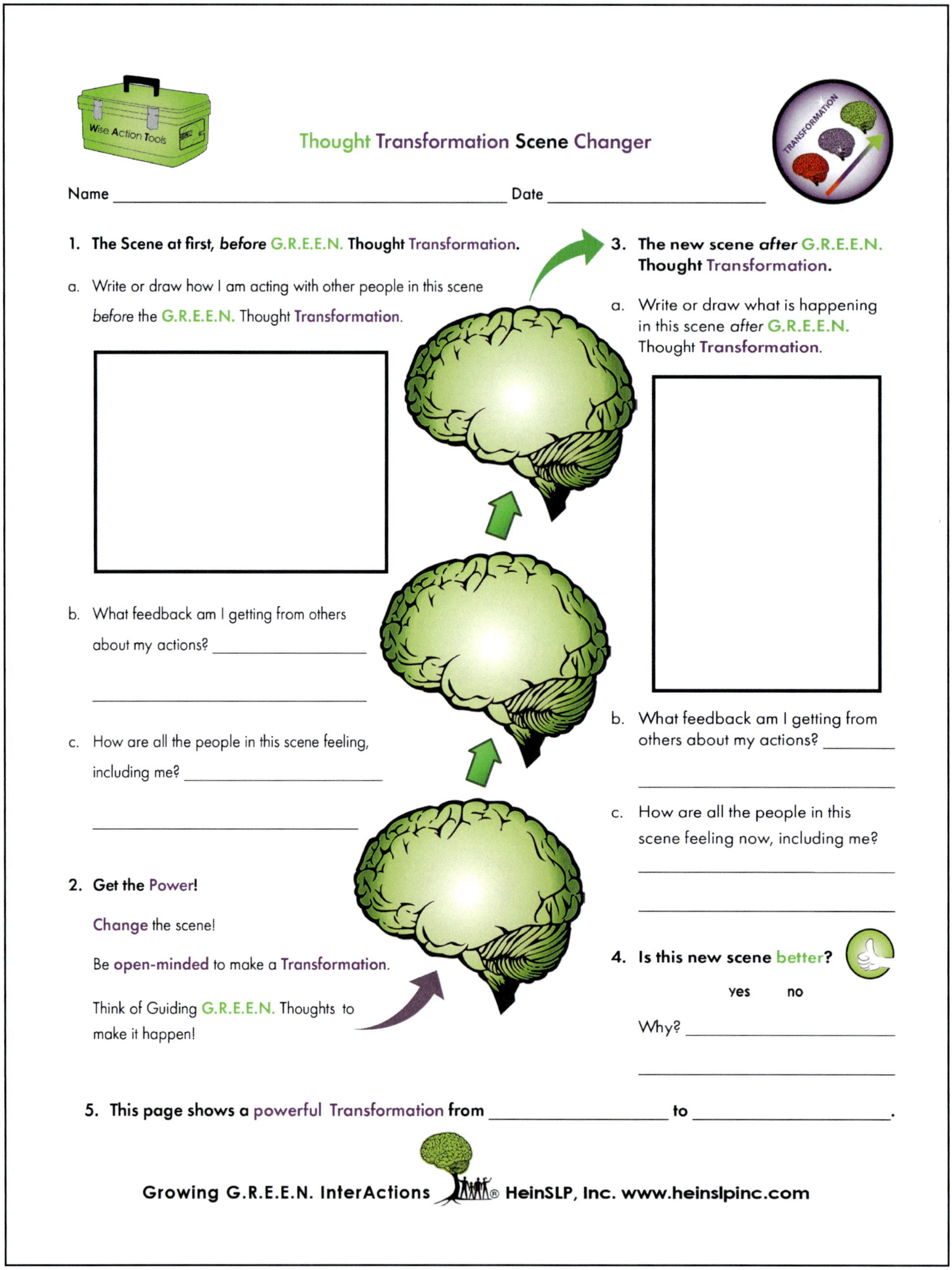

Thought Transformation Scene Changer

Name ______________________ Date ______________

1. **The Scene at first, *before* G.R.E.E.N. Thought Transformation.**

a. Write or draw how I am acting with other people in this scene *before* the G.R.E.E.N. Thought **Transformation**.

b. What feedback am I getting from others about my actions? ______________

____

c. How are all the people in this scene feeling, including me? ______________

____

2. **Get the Power!**

Change the scene!

Be **open-minded** to make a **Transformation**.

Think of Guiding G.R.E.E.N. Thoughts to make it happen!

3. **The new scene *after* G.R.E.E.N. Thought Transformation.**

a. Write or draw what is happening in this scene *after* G.R.E.E.N. Thought **Transformation**.

b. What feedback am I getting from others about my actions? ______________

____

c. How are all the people in this scene feeling now, including me?

____

____

4. **Is this new scene better?**

yes no

Why? ______________

____

5. **This page shows a powerful Transformation from ______________ to ______________.**

Growing G.R.E.E.N. InterActions® HeinSLP, Inc. www.heinslpinc.com

Figure 14. Thought Transformation Scene Changer worksheet

4.16 Becoming Aware of Mixed Feelings and Being Positive on the Outside

This program encourages participants to make **transformations** so they can make situations better for themselves and those around them. Strategies are available to assist them if they have mixed feelings, both **positive** and negative. In the section of the ***Lesson Book*** titled "**Being Easygoing When You Have Mixed Feelings**," participants are guided to think about and draw how the scene would look if they acted on their negative feelings. They also are guided to include the important element of how those around them would act and feel as a consequence of their negative actions. They then are guided to repeat the exercise, this time thinking and drawing the scene that would result from acting on **positive** feelings, again indicating how others would act and feel. They then are encouraged to cover up the negative picture, keeping those feelings and related actions on the "inside." Instead, they are guided to focus on the picture of **positive** action that they drew. Following through on showing these actions and feelings on the "outside" would benefit everyone on their Team (Figure 15). Participants can be encouraged to feel pride when they can transform themselves to have the self-control needed to only show their "outside" actions.

4.17 You Are a Work in Progress and Have a Second Chance to Act Even Better

We are not perfect. We are human. We can learn from our mistakes. Guides can help participants believe this by having the attitude, modeling the attitude, and teaching the attitude that we can do better when given another chance to act.

Participants are usually motivated to act out **G.R.E.E.N. Scenes** and to act them out more than once. Then they are usually more willing to take advice in these structured situations, resulting in increasingly more prosocial and **G.R.E.E.N.** actions. They will sense that they don't have to be perfect the first time they are allowed a second opportunity to role-play. They become better at accepting the support provided for them to act better when given another opportunity. They begin to learn that we can always do things to make a scene even better. They can then benefit from discussion regarding how their improved action led to **positive** consequences, benefiting their character, their Team, and **Common Team Goal** (Figure 16).

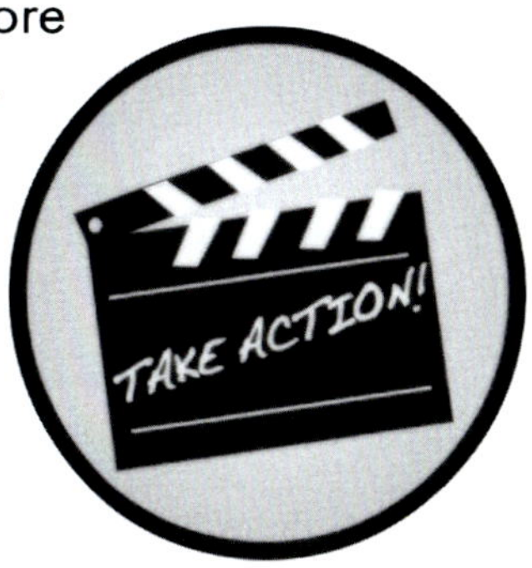

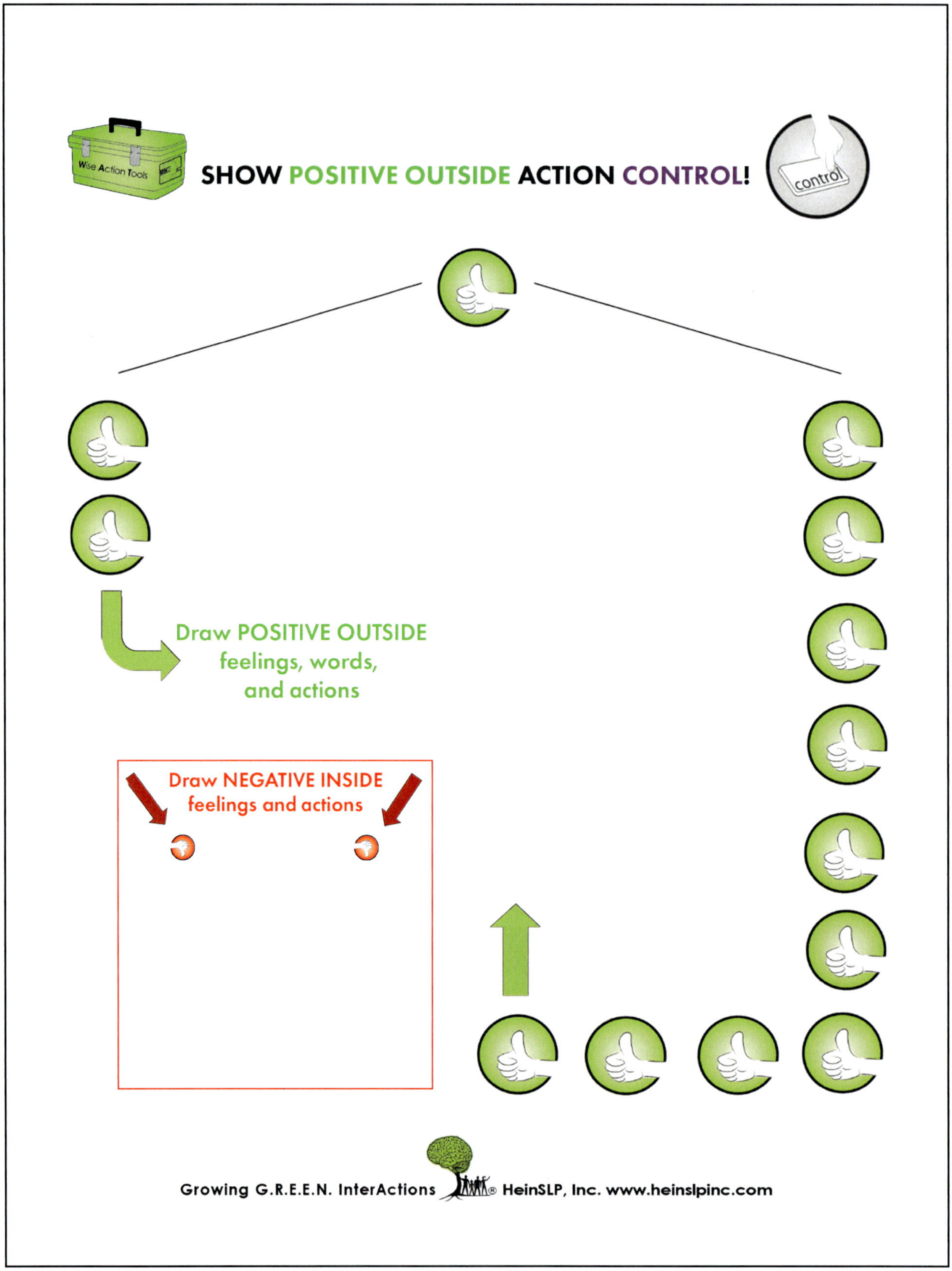

Figure 15. Show Positive Outside Action Control! worksheet

G.R.E.E.N. SCENE REVIEW FORM

Date ______________________ Name of Reviewer ______________________

Name of G.R.E.E.N. Scene/Situation ______________________

The goal of this "Team" ______________________

G.R.E.E.N. SCENE TEAM MEMBER	ROLE IN THIS SCENE	G Grateful said "thank you" or otherwise showed appreciation	R Respectful used polite words and tone of voice	E Empathetic acted as if they cared about the other people	E Easygoing acted cooperatively to help achieve the TEAM goal	N Navigating stayed calm and handled a challenging situation
1.						
2.						
3.						

Comments—extra "takes" or cues needed? ______________________

Growing G.R.E.E.N. InterActions® HeinSLP, Inc. www.heinslpinc.com

Figure 16. G.R.E.E.N. Scene Review Form

4.18 Listening to and Respectfully Conversing with People Who Have Different Interests and Points of View

The **Growing G.R.E.E.N. InterActions Program** presents lessons and activities to teach participants about points of view other than their own, and that learning other points of view can be extremely valuable. Mutually beneficial action can then be taken that considers more than one point of view. Emphasis is also placed on teaching participants that different people have different interests. People are considered respectful and easygoing when they take time to talk about another person's topic of interest and learn about it.

This program guides participants to stay on the **Conversation Team Topic**, especially when it is about the other person's topic of interest (Figure 17).

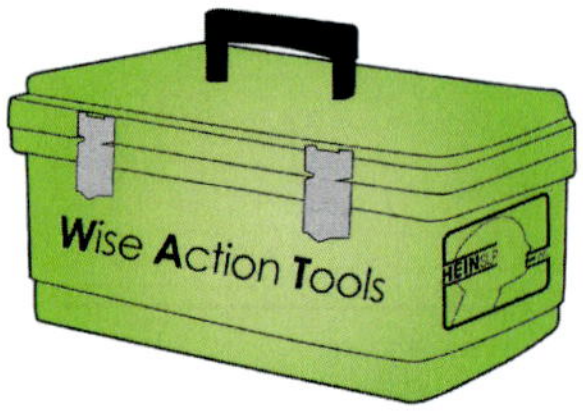

ON-TOPIC TRACKER

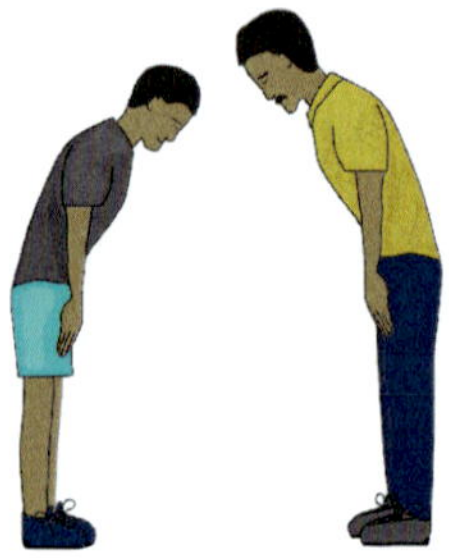

1. What is this Conversation Team Topic? ______________________________

____

2. Fill in the names of the conversation partners and check when each partner asks a question or makes a comment that relates to the Team topic. Check on the bottom if each partner stayed **on-topic** or went off-topic during this conversation.

______________ CONVERSATION PARTNER #1	______________ CONVERSATION PARTNER #2
____ **question(s) asked about the Team topic** __ __ __ __ __	____ **question(s) asked about the Team topic** __ __ __ __ __
____ **comments made about the Team topic** __ __ __ __ __	____ **comments made about the Team topic** __ __ __ __ __
ON-TOPIC OFF-TOPIC	ON-TOPIC OFF-TOPIC

3. Did both conversation partners stay **on-topic**? yes no

4. After both conversation partners have stayed **on-topic** about one topic, they can start to have another **on-topic** conversation about a different topic.

Figure 17. On-Topic Tracker worksheet

After participants learn what it means to stay on a common topic, the guide can use the **Topics for Caring Conversations** worksheet (Figure 18) to help participants keep track of their **conversational** partners' topics of interest. Participants then can be guided to engage in conversation about their **conversational** partner's preferred topic.

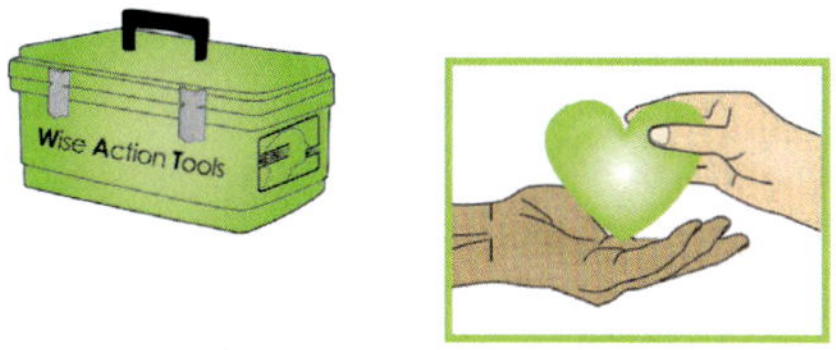

TOPICS FOR CARING CONVERSATIONS

I care about these people, so I keep track of the topics they care about. I can show I care by talking about these topics in my conversations with them.

Person I Care About	This Person Cares About These Topics

Growing G.R.E.E.N. InterActions® HeinSLP, Inc. www.heinslpinc.com

Figure 18. Topics for Caring Conversations worksheet

Using visual aids from the **Wise Action Tool** called **Building My Conversation Power by Paying Attention, Asking Questions & Taking Notes** (Figure 19), participants learn to listen when people are talking about their topics of interest and make comments and ask questions about these topics even when they were initially "nonpreferred." Participants learn to focus on nonpreferred topics by taking notes about them. Eventually participants learn to perceive and respond to the topic without using notes.

BUILDING MY CONVERSATION POWER BY PAYING ATTENTION, ASKING QUESTIONS & TAKING NOTES

1A. I AM TALKING TO ______________________ Date ______________

1B. I CHOOSE A TOPIC: This is a topic that I think this person would like to talk about today: ______

____

2. I ASK A QUESTION: I ask a question to learn something new about the topic:

   How is ______________________________________?

   or *Tell me what's new with* ______________________________

3. I LISTEN AND TAKE NOTES: I use my power to listen carefully and write down an important detail about what was said: ______________________________

____

4. I MAKE A COMMENT: (*Wow! That's interesting! That's great! Sounds good! Too bad.)* ______

____

5. I ASK A RELATED QUESTION: I ask another question about what the person just said: .

   How do you feel about ______________________________?

   Can you tell me more about ___________________________?

   What __________? *Where* __________? *Why* __________?

6. I LISTEN AND TAKE NOTES: I use my power to listen carefully and write down an important detail about what was said: ______________________________

____

7. I MAKE A FINAL COMMENT THAT SHOWS I WAS LISTENING TO WHAT THE PERSON SAID:
   I politely end the conversation by saying one or more of the following:

   That's very interesting! Thanks for telling me about ____________________

   I'm glad that ______________________________

   or I'm sorry that ______________________________

   and I hope that ______________________________

(When we are done talking, I can draw a detailed picture to help me remember what my conversation partner said about this topic.)

Figure 19. Building My Conversation Power worksheet

The participant also learns to interact and engage in respectful conversation by becoming more aware of the need to monitor topic choices. They learn to be aware of the categories on the **Hein Conversational Rating Scale** (Figure 20) to avoid offending or startling their conversation partners or anyone else in the scene. They learn to appreciate the positive consequences of *gaining* social points rather than *losing* them.

The participant also learns to interact and engage in respectful conversation by becoming more aware of the need to monitor topic choices. They learn to be aware of the categories on the **Hein Conversational Rating Scale** (Figure 20) to avoid offending or startling their conversation partners or anyone else in the scene. They learn to appreciate the positive consequences of *gaining* social points rather than *losing* them.

Wise Action Tools

HEIN CONVERSATIONAL RATING SCALE

I have to think about:

- my choice of topic and if it is appropriate for my audience
- my choice of words and if they are appropriate for my audience
- my tone of voice
- my audience
- how much humor/teasing I can safely use with my audience and still be taken seriously when needed

G = General Audiences—What I say would be OK with Grandma or the school principal. I am on topic and am not saying anything odd, strange, mean, disgusting, or violent. No swear words are used at all. I get a lot of social points for being able to control my topic and my words. I am considered mature.

PG = Possible Guidance needed—What I want to say may be slightly funny or sarcastic. I need to know if my audience will appreciate my topic and words without my losing social points. With this style, I might be considered immature.

R = Restricted—The topic and word choice would offend most people. I can use this language only at special times with people who would appreciate my odd, strange, mean, disgusting, or violent topics. If I use this language in class or public, I will get in trouble and lose many social points. People will not trust that I can control myself and I will lose privileges and responsibilities. I should avoid saying things that are really off topic because people will consider them R-rated and will not want to have conversations with me in the future.

X = eXtremely Limited—These topics and words are so inappropriate, strange, odd, violent, disgusting, or mean that they really should not be said out loud. I should limit even thinking about these topics or words. Most people will be extremely offended, upset, or worried if they hear these words or topics, and I will get in serious trouble and lose all my social points.

Growing G.R.E.E.N. InterActions® HeinSLP, Inc. www.heinslpinc.com

Figure 20. Hein Conversational Rating Scale

4.19 Cooperative Conversations and Compromises

The framework provided in the Cooperative Conversation **Ingredients Checklist** (Figure 21) assists participants in clearly perceiving the critical elements involved in a Cooperative Conversation. Guides can help participants determine what the conversation is about (**Situation Topic**) and what goal both conversation partners are striving to accomplish (Common Team Goal).

Participants can then judge whether conversations found in the *Interactive* ***Lesson Book*** have all the following "ingredients" of a Cooperative Conversation:

Did both people have a chance to tell what they wanted or needed?

Did both people listen to find out what the other person wanted?

Did both people work together to find a way to have each other's needs met?

If all ingredients were included, the conversation was cooperative. If not, participants are guided to find what was missing in order to make the next conversation more cooperative.

If there is an opportunity to lead two participants through a cooperative conversation, the guide can help them answer critical questions ahead of time. Guides can help participants determine and "name" what the conversation is about (**Situation Topic**) to keep it focused and action-oriented. They can also help participants determine a goal both conversation partners can agree that they are striving to accomplish (Common Team Goal).

The guide can help participants in the conversation ask the types of questions noted below to clarify the **Situation Topic**:

What do we need to figure out together in this conversation?

Here are some examples of sentence starters for some typical things people need to figure out when having cooperative conversations:

How do we share . . . ?

Why do we need . . . ?

How do we make . . . ?

Where do we put . . . ?

When do we go . . . ?

The guide can help participants answer questions that will help them determine a **Common Team Goal** that both conversation partners can agree on such as:

What is something we both agree we would want to accomplish in this conversation?

Here is an example of a **Common Team Goal** that works in most cases:

We will understand the situation from both points of view and work things out so we both feel satisfied with our plan.

The participants will then be able to engage in a conversation, filling out the **Cooperative Conversation Ingredients Checklist** when done to see if the necessary conversation elements were included. They can be guided to have a more cooperative conversation the next time they speak with each other, making sure to add in any missing "ingredients."

Lessons and activities are included that teach participants about the elements of **compromise** and whether specific situations call for it. They learn that in a **compromise** neither side gets everything they want, but both sides get some needs met so they can move **forward**.

Each person involved in a **compromise** can say, "If I do this, then you will do that." Each side must follow-through on what they say they will do (Figure 22).

Participants also learn that some situations become safer and better for the whole Team when its members do just what is asked without needing to engage in a **compromise** process. In such situations, not spending time and effort to make a **compromise** becomes a better choice for the whole Team.

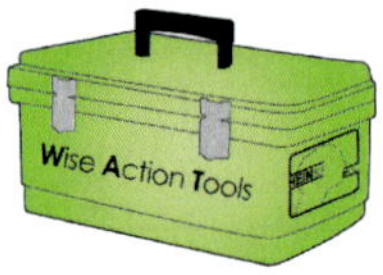

WORKSHEET FOR MAKING A G.R.E.E.N. TEAM COMPROMISE

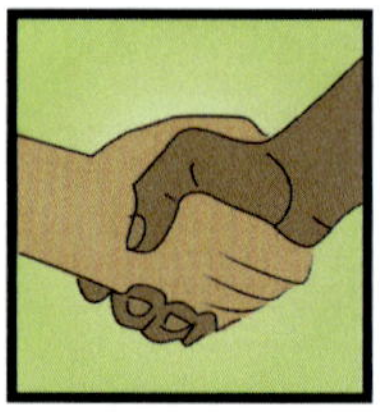

Here is the situation that needs a Team compromise:

____

____

____

Our Shared G.R.E.E.N. Compromise:

This is the G.R.E.E.N. compromise we have made together.

We both get some needs met so we can both move forward.

If I ____

____

then you ____

____

If you ____

____

then I ____

____

Figure 21. Team Compromise worksheet

COOPERATIVE CONVERSATION INGREDIENTS CHECKLIST

Name ______________________________ Date ____________________

Think about the ingredients needed in a Cooperative Conversation. Mark this checklist to show whether Persons #1 and #2 have included those ingredients.

Situation Topic: ____

____

Common Team Goal ____

____

Ingredients for a Cooperative Conversation	Name of Person #1: ____________	Name of Person #2: ____________	Did both people work cooperatively?
1. Calmly and respectfully *tell* what each person needs.	Did this person calmly and respecttfully use words to say what was needed? yes no	Did this person calmly and respecttfully use words to say what was needed? yes no	Did both people have a chance to *tell* what they wanted or needed? yes no
2. Respectfully and patiently listen to what each person needs.	Did this person respectfully and patiently listen to what the other person needed? yes no	Did this person respectfully and patiently listen to what the other person needed? yes no	Did both people listen to find out what the other person wanted or needed? yes no
3. Respectfully and **patiently** use words to *share ideas, making a plan* to meet *both* people's needs. Both people win!	Did this person say something to help the other person feel that their needs will be met? yes no	Did this person say something to help the other person feel that their needs will be met? yes no	Did both pople work together to flexibly find a way to meet each other's needs? yes no

Are all ingredients included? yes no

If not, circle the ingredients to add to make the next conversation more cooperative.

Figure 22. Cooperative Conversation Ingredients Checklist

5 Important Considerations for the Guiding of Program Participants

5.1 Powerful Guidance Helps Others Make Transformations

"I can't do anything to help this person."

"This situation will never change."

Or ➡ "I believe I can help this person understand this situation in a different way so a **positive** behavioral **transformation** can occur."

It is important that guides believe that the way they provide instruction helps reframe participant perceptions about experiences. Your approaches can **transform** the participant's perception of an experience!

5.2 Using Self-Awareness to Make the Best Action Choices

"This will never work. This person does not care about acting well and will always act in a negative way."

Or ➡ "This will work!"

➡ "I can provide clues so this person becomes more aware of their actions and makes the best action choices independently."

Often, teachers, therapists, and parents believe that certain individuals are incapable of being aware of their behavior. My experience has been that when we patiently present essential tools at the most fundamental level, individuals can perceive, practice, and ultimately experience the benefits of self-monitoring and self-control strategies. I have found that language, music, and self-calming strategies help individuals access a calmer state. With these **powerful** tools, participants can then learn to assert themselves by expressing their wants, needs, and concerns effectively. Actively practicing these self-calming approaches and scripts for appropriate assertiveness can guide participants to make their situations better for themselves and others.

Building on this concept, **Growing G.R.E.E.N. InterActions** encourages individuals to use self-control strategies by explicitly providing the language and clear step-by-step explanations of how and when to use these strategies.

It is critical to realize that those we are guiding can sense when we have given up on them. Therefore, for **positive** changes to be made, we as guides must do our best to keep **positive** thoughts in our minds:

> *These people can* **transform** *their behavior.*
>
> *It will just take more time, or I need to change something in my approach.*

5.3 Providing Explicit Instructions to Participants

> "This person does not know how to act at all. She said to me, 'You are telling me to do it, but I don't know how. If I did, I would be doing it already!' "

Or ➡ "Wow! If I provide more support and show exactly what I want said or done, this person can start doing it!"

Having worked collaboratively as the speech-language pathologist in private special education schools, as the classroom teacher of communicatively handicapped students in the public schools, and as the provider of functional treatment to brain-injured individuals of all ages, I realized that my materials and my instruction need to be explicit. I have attended lectures presented by author-educator Anita Archer, a proponent of the importance of explicit instruction in the field of education. She has seen the benefits of providing systematic, direct, engaging, and success-oriented instruction. She believes in the necessity of modeling the behavior to be taught before expecting students to perform successfully on their own.

These program materials clearly present information to participants by

1. Defining vocabulary that may be unfamiliar
2. Clearly explaining all concepts
3. Providing relevant examples of the concepts presented

To be as clear as possible, choices of what to think, say, and do are also explicitly presented. This allows participants to feel confident in knowing exactly what to say in the presented situations, and feel successful in their interactions as a result. When given such explicit choices, the perception of their behavior as successfully prosocial and G.R.E.E.N. becomes more likely. Guides can continue to provide explicit instruction to participants as needed to help them in their real-life interactions.

5.4 Providing Activities at the Right Level

Participants might say:

"This is too hard for me to understand."

"You are going way too fast!"

"I don't feel like I can be successful at all!"

Or

- "I understand what you are talking about."
- "You are explaining things as you go along at a rate that I can process and understand."
- "I feel successful. I am learning."

Activities should be presented at a rate and complexity that allow participants to perform successfully with minimal coaching. Continue checking to see whether you are presenting information at the right level and adjust your presentation to make it easier or harder as needed.

In individual sessions (compared with group or whole-classroom instruction), it is easier to select and present these materials to match the participant.

As guides, we should ask ourselves:

- How much am I presenting at one time?
- How quickly am I presenting this information?
- How complex is this information?
- How often do I need to repeat what I already presented?
- How much time can I spend on one activity to maintain the participant's best attention?

The materials provided in this program can be used at different levels to allow for greater individualization based on individual needs.

Some program aspects may be too difficult for a participant to understand or master. In such cases, a more fundamental aspect of the concept could be presented instead.

We don't expect each participant to perform at the same level. Consider the following progression of instruction:

1. To provide the most assistance, we can model an exact answer and have the participant repeat it, or point to a printed version of it.
2. We can expect a participant to select from a choice of answers.
3. We can expect a participant to spontaneously give an answer if the information has already been taught.
4. To challenge participants who need the material to be more complex, relevant, or challenging, we can ask them why they have chosen a particular answer.
5. We can ask whether participants have had a similar personal experience in order to expand the discussion.

In group situations, the main lesson can be chosen with different participants engaged in different aspects of the material. Some participants can be guided to respond at more basic levels, and some can expand and make personal connections.

In a classroom setting, some responses from the stronger participants can be written on the board, with other participants choosing one or more of the written answers when responding.

As a guide, you may need to model every response and have participants repeat what was modeled. Some participants will require multiple repetitions to understand and begin using the concepts.

Using a Team Approach

"I am separate."

"I don't think of myself as part of the same group."

"It is them against me."

Or ➡ "We are all part of a Team."

➡ "We work together so the Team becomes better."

A key aspect of this program is its focus on developing a Team approach. No matter whether a Home, Classroom, or Friendship Team, we are on a Team and the Team has certain goals that it wants to achieve.

Choose words that develop a Team focus. In contrast to the more typical conversation about what you did right or wrong versus what I did, the focus can be on what *we* are doing together for *us*, the *Team*. This encourages more self-motivated, **positive** action, as fewer authoritarian commands are presented that appear to be unclear and arbitrary. Instead, more collaborative action and joint acknowledgment of how the Team is moving **forward** can be achieved.

This focus on the Team encourages participants to make their best efforts to help the Team. This sets up a unified front, in contrast to the language of "you" versus "me" that creates a scene with opposing sides.

Model and rehearse Team-centered awareness. Thinking of their Team does not come naturally to those who are primarily focused only on their own needs. This may happen in cases of neurological differences, in which individuals lack the "mirror neurons" needed to perceive what others are feeling. It also does not come naturally to some people with emotional challenges whose imbalances in brain chemistry may make it difficult for them to match their behavior to the social situations in which they find themselves. However, I have found that through modeling and rehearsing scenes and presenting language focused on the Team's needs and actions, people with high-level autism and those with emotional disturbances can successfully learn to pay more attention to Team activities. The resulting changes in behavior then benefit the Team.

Expand the Team-centered concept for the general population. Many features of our current culture encourage individuals to be concerned primarily with their own welfare. Without a cultural force concerned with people besides ourselves, actions are frequently taken without concern for how they affect others. For example, drivers frequently change lanes without signaling; it appears that these people are not concerned with the welfare of others on the road, and do not consider the **Common Team Goal** that everyone arrives safely at their destination.

To counteract this, a concerted effort should be made to consider everyone on a common road and common Team with each driver thinking the following **Guiding G.R.E.E.N. Thought**:

> *"I need to communicate my movements to someone out there besides me, especially if I am moving into another person's space."*

The key idea to develop is that the individual benefits along with the group when Team-centered actions take place. Whenever possible, this message of acting in a mutually beneficial manner, and recognizing that others are on the same Team, needs to go out to those for whom this kind of awareness and thinking are limited. The idea of being on the same Team in different situations is quite **powerful**. We can start to guide our students, clients, and children to be more Team-focused in most situations, particularly because our society may not always be providing healthy modeling for developing this kind of Team awareness.

5.5 Highlight and Reinforce Actions for Team Goals While Supporting Attainment of Personal Goals

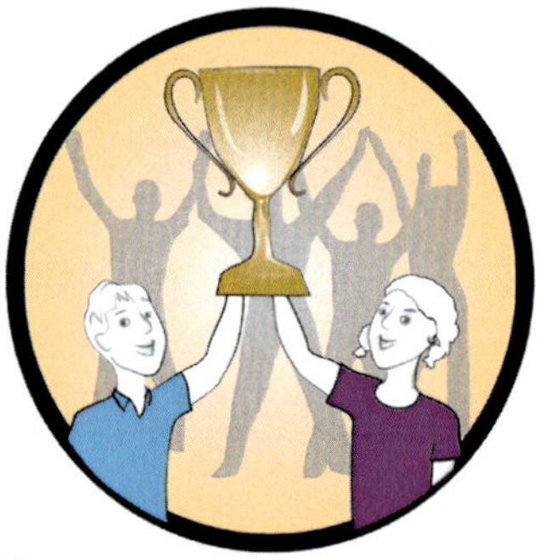

"I don't have anything in common with this person."

"I don't even pay attention to this other person."

"We are following our own path and nothing intersects."

Or

- "I pay attention to you because we are on the same Team."
- "We both have at least one goal in common."
- "We can do what we need to do to meet our **Common Team Goal**."
- "Helping the Team meet the **Common Team Goal** will probably help each of us meet our **Personal Goals**, too."

A. Explicitly spell out and consistently support at least one Common Team Goal.

The **Growing G.R.E.E.N. InterActions Program** heavily stresses that participants are always on a Team no matter whom they are with, and integrates the idea that everyone can work to support at least one Common Team Goal. Guides can help Team members engage in discussion using the following:

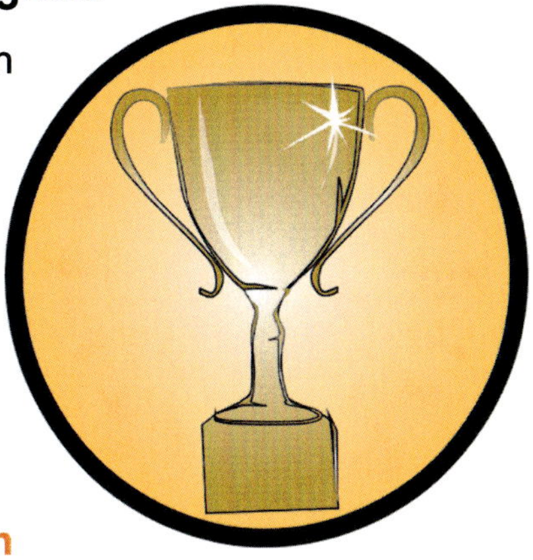

"If we can figure out and name our Common Team Goal, we will become more aware of it, act on it, stick to it and achieve it!"

Everyone's behavior improves as Team members experience the support they give others while others in turn support them.

The important question to ask in a situation is, "What's our Common Team Goal?"

B. Encourage the development of Personal Goals that are aligned with Common Team Goals.

The ***Lesson Book*** includes a section encouraging participants to choose and write their Personal Goals. Establishment of clear-cut goals for individuals and groups helps direct their daily attention to moving closer to those goals.

If we don't name our direction, we will experience difficulty with consistently moving toward it. Guiding participants to become aware of Personal and Common Team Goals and repeatedly state them has been comforting and helpful within this program. With the reinforcement of the Personal and Common Team Goals, most participants can increase on-task behaviors and productivity, knowing that they are on a supportive Team.

5.6 The Effect of Individual Behavior on the Team

"She has no idea how her actions affect others and doesn't seem to care."

"He does what he wants because he does not realize he is part of a group."

Or ➡ "She is more aware of the others on her Team right now and is starting to pay attention to whether she is helping the Team."

➡ "Because he is now thinking of the Team, he is taking his time to Think First before acting. He is making choices to really help the Team meet its goal of making the classroom a safe place for everyone to learn."

This program highlights the effects of individual behavior on movement toward achieving **Common Team Goals**. Instead of focusing on a particular behavior's **positive** and negative effects on individual people, the program focuses on how individual behavior affects Teams. This broadens participants' awareness of their effects on the group. Participants often are less reactive to receiving Team-related feedback as a result. The following feedback examples use Team terminology:

"Your actions are really helping the Team."

"Are your actions helping the Team *right now?"*

"Let's think about what you can do to help the Team *right now."*

"Let's remember the **Common Team Goal** and *determine the changes we can make to help meet it."*

5.7 Be Relevant

This person is getting off task and asking, "What does this have to do with me? This has nothing to do with my life."

Or ➡ "This person is giving me his full attention and saying, 'I see how this can be useful for me in my life.' "

Providing relevant and meaningful instructional material is also important for **Growing G.R.E.E.N. InterActions**. After laying out the program's basic foundational concepts, the guide can select the scenes most relevant for the needs of participants. Also, participants can be encouraged to connect the lessons, concepts, and strategies to their lives. After the target behavior has been presented and participants have been guided to practice it within structured activities, they can be encouraged to generate guiding thoughts and individual scripts for related scenes. Promoting individualization of appropriate responses allows the material to be personally relevant and increases the likelihood that this new behavior will be carried over to real-life situations. Through this approach, the concepts and strategies of the program's scenarios and scripts will become embedded within each participant's experiences.

5.8 Be Empowering

The student thinks, *This doesn't make me feel like I have any control*!

Or ➡ *I feel like I have control over this scene to make it better. I have tools that I can use to make my life better.*

This program strongly emphasizes the harnessing of **power** by participants using their human brains to make the best choices. Frequently, children and even some adults feel that they do not have control over themselves and what they do. Through this program, these individuals can be guided to begin to gain some of that **power** over themselves and their actions.

To guide personal **empowerment**, participants are first given opportunities to practice obtaining the self-control they need. Then they are guided to select the personally relevant **Guiding G.R.E.E.N. Thoughts** that can help them make the best **G.R.E.E.N.** choices in their real lives. Participants learn that they have the **power** to ask for what they need and do what is needed to make their life scenes more effective and successful.

Through the guided opportunities to make **positive** action choices and choose **G.R.E.E.N.** words that benefit the Team, participants start to experience what it feels like to affect others in a **positive** way. They begin to feel how **powerful** it can be to have self-control, allowing them to **transform** as needed, by guiding their thoughts and actions, to benefit whatever Team they are with.

5.9 Guide Self-Assessment and Provide Frequent Reinforcement to Shape Desired Behavior

"He always is doing the wrong thing."

"I can't do anything to change her behavior."

"I know he won't behave in the right way."

Or

- "There are times when he does something close to what I want him to do, and I reinforce that behavior.
- "I catch her when she is on target and reinforce her actions as much as she can tolerate."
- "I let him know exactly what he was doing that showed me he was making good choices and acting G.R.E.E.N.!"

As human beings, we make the most gains when we receive reinforcement for staying on track and taking steps **forward**. This also is true for participants of this program. Through the reinforcements embedded within the **Growing G.R.E.E.N. InterActions Program**, participants receive **positive** feedback when they Think First and make prosocial choices that benefit themselves and their Teams. They experience the **positive** consequences of prosocial behavior in structured activities, and then that behavior is reinforced further with the **G.R.E.E.N. Actions Evaluation** worksheet (first introduced as Figure 6) as they attempt to carry over G.R.E.E.N. actions into their classrooms, homes, friendships, and communities.

A. Provide baseline and ongoing self-assessments and opportunities for participants to review others' assessments of their G.R.E.E.N. functioning

Participants have the opportunity to evaluate themselves on how frequently they display G.R.E.E.N. behavior. They then reevaluate themselves periodically. As they acquire prosocial behavior and practice it in structured situations, they can see whether they have been realistic and honest with themselves. It is also possible to share with them how other people on their Teams view their G.R.E.E.N. behavior when their teachers, therapists, and parents complete the same evaluation form. As they learn about the value of being on a Team, they can learn to value the opinion of others on their Team and to accept the constructive feedback from others.

Participants are encouraged to perceive and reinforce G.R.E.E.N. behavior not only in themselves, but also when shown by others on their Teams. This encourages attention to the target behaviors in Team members and encourages demonstrating their support of others. The **Wise Action Tool** called the **G.R.E.E.N. Actions Evaluation Chart** can be used for participant self-assessment and G.R.E.E.N. evaluations by others. Participants can compare their grand totals over time and be guided to see differences between their self-assessments and the assessment feedback of others.

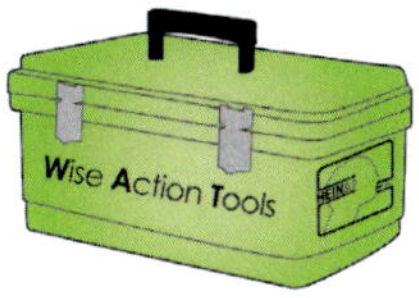

G.R.E.E.N. ACTIONS EVALUATION CHART

Team Member: ______________________ Today's Date ____________

Evaluation by:

- ☐ Self
- ☐ Teacher
- ☐ Parent
- ☐ Peer
- ☐ Other ____________

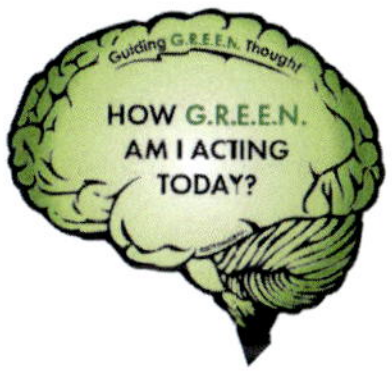

HONESTLY EVALUATE ACTIONS BY CHECKING THE BOX THAT IS TRUE TODAY

	NEVER 0	A LITTLE BIT 1	HALF THE TIME 2	MOST OF THE TIME 3	ALL THE TIME 4	TOTAL
GRATEFUL- I let people know that I appreciate what I have.						
RESPECTFUL- I am respectful of the people and things in every situation. I use a tone of voice that is positive and polite.						
EMPATHETIC- I show that I am considerate of the feelings of my friends, classmates, and family.						
EASYGOING- I am open-minded and cooperate with people to meet Team goals.						
NAVIGATING- I am flexible when I manage challenges because I stay calm and make wise choices.						
I take responsibility for my actions and accept consequences.						
				GRAND TOTAL		

Growing G.R.E.E.N. InterActions® HeinSLP, Inc. www.heinslpinc.com

B. **Provide motivating and relevant rewards for participation**

Choose motivating rewards relevant to participants. Initially, participants can be given a tangible token to reinforce prosocial behavior. The **G.R.E.E.N. Token Tracker** can help the instructor keep the student engaged during a lesson. Depending on the age of participants, a small tangible prize can be given to each participant who accumulates five tokens per lesson. The achievement of on-task behaviors can be integrated into classroom reward systems. When students are rewarded, other students are encouraged to give verbal praise, which provides additional motivation for everyone to earn their five tokens.

Reward systems can be established within Classroom and Home Teams. Check marks on charts can be totaled, and prizes or privileges can be bestowed at Classroom and Home reinforcement meetings.

C. **Use tracking and reinforcement tools as participants act G.R.E.E.N. to increase the frequency of positive actions.**

Several tracking and reinforcement tools are provided in this program, and their use is explained in this section. Guides should implement these tools in partnership with their participants. Most are "**Wise Action Tools**" that can be kept in folders, and Team members can access them in the classroom or home. Several tools reinforce positive actions:

- **G.R.E.E.N. Token Tracker** for maintaining attention and participation in lessons
- **G.R.E.E.N. Action Report** for noting observed G.R.E.E.N. behavior that occurs during the day so the participant gets "credit" for the prosocial action
- My Personal **G.R.E.E.N. Action Tracker** for participants to track the amount of G.R.E.E.N. action they exhibited during a week
- **G.R.E.E.N. Action Tracker** for the Classroom Team for the Classroom Guide to track Classroom Team progress
- **G.R.E.E.N. Action Tracker** for the Home Team for the Home Guide to track Home Team progress

G.R.E.E.N. Token Tracker

Each participant receives a **G.R.E.E.N. Token Tracker** (first introduced as Figure 1) at the beginning of each lesson. Participants are told that they will be rewarded for maintaining attention and participating throughout the session. The guide gives out five tokens to each participant, one at a time, as they show the target behavior. Participant actions are immediately reinforced whenever **G.R.E.E.N.** behavior is independently demonstrated. The goals of this system are to maintain attention within the therapy room or classroom and immediately reinforce targeted behaviors. The Token Tracker gives participants a visual cue reminding them that the immediate goal is achieving a targeted behavior at least five times during the lesson. Having the Token Tracker in front of them reminds participants to monitor their behavior, and it further motivates them to maintain attention and on-target behavior throughout the lesson.

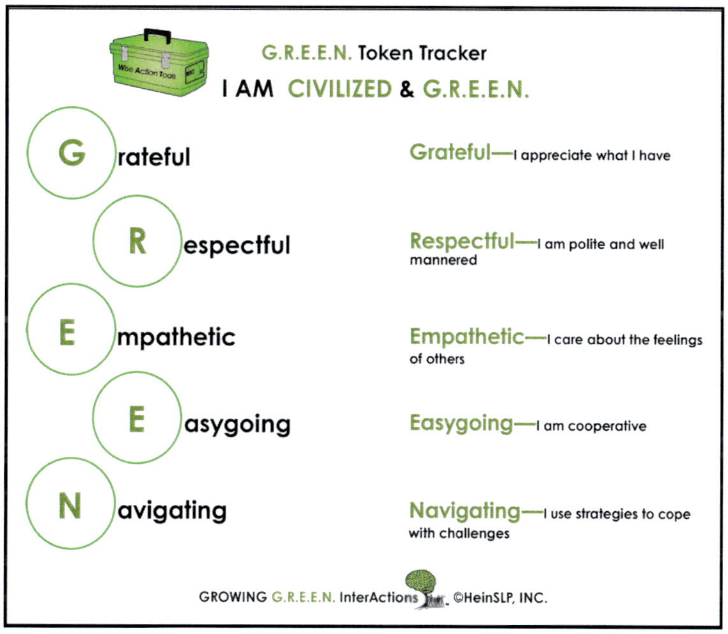

Tokens may be distributed with less delay to those participants who need continual reinforcement or are not skilled at "delaying gratification." Gradually the guide can encourage participants to maintain on-task **G.R.E.E.N.** behavior with less need for immediate feedback.

To encourage self-control, the "rule" is that the green tokens must stay on the card and cannot fall on the floor if they are to be counted at the end of the lesson. If the participant breaks this rule, the guide can emphasize that the participant will have more opportunities in the near future to show increased self-control.

A guide might provide these instructions:

> *"I am going to hand out your Token Trackers for today's lesson. Keep them on your desks in the best location for carefully placing your tokens on the* **G.R.E.E.N.** *letters."*
>
> *"If a green token is in each circle by the end of the lesson and none have fallen on the floor, the reward will be ____________________________. All of you are doing a great job on this Class Team, so let's keep it going."*

Younger participants and those less able to wait to be rewarded on another day should receive a tangible reward at the end of each session. Eventually these tangible reinforcers can be reduced in amount and frequency. Often the Token Tracker becomes no longer necessary, because students have learned sufficient self-control and do not need extrinsic reinforcement to pay attention to the lesson. Students can learn to be internally motivated to act **G.R.E.E.N.** as they realize this kind of action makes their lives better.

G.R.E.E.N. Action Report—Detailed Positive Reinforcement Notes

The **G.R.E.E.N. Action Report** (first introduced as Figure 8) encourages guides to engage in the critically important step of reinforcing participant behavior whenever participants are caught acting **G.R.E.E.N.**! Participants can initially be reinforced with these **G.R.E.E.N. Action Reports** for displaying any respectful, easygoing, cooperative behavior in any interaction with the guide, especially when the guide is presenting structured lessons. For those new to exhibiting **G.R.E.E.N.** behaviors, any approximations of prosocial behavior can be reinforced. A guide can fill out a **G.R.E.E.N. Action Report** and give it to a participant any time these skills begin to be exhibited in less structured situations. With this note, the participant is given credit for spontaneously acting in the new, improved way. As appropriate, the guide can make the reinforcement even stronger by discussing the positive action with the participant while filling out the form. These notes can eventually help participants think independently about being **G.R.E.E.N.** all day.

This important program element focuses participant attention on acting G.R.E.E.N. while also noticing the G.R.E.E.N. action of others. When eliciting G.R.E.E.N. behavior within a Team, Team members can be guided to reinforce one another's positive behavior, first in structured and then in unstructured situations. At first, the guide can take the time to teach participants how to fill out G.R.E.E.N. **Action Reports**. Then a structured activity can be set up for participants to be assisted in filling these out to reinforce any G.R.E.E.N. behavior they noticed other Team members display. Relevant scripts in the program provide modeling of G.R.E.E.N. behaviors that participants act out. This enables them to recognize similar behavior as it occurs within their own Team interactions. Particularly useful is guiding participants to notice when their Teammates display any of the specific behaviors discussed and practiced in the most recent lessons and G.R.E.E.N. **scenes**. Eventually, participants learn to initiate completing detailed G.R.E.E.N. **Action Reports** on their own.

In addition to having participants write their notes, it is equally important to set aside time to share these notes with the group. The G.R.E.E.N. notes can be kept in a G.R.E.E.N. box made by some members of the Classroom Team. The notes can then be read at a particular time of the day or week. As the notes are read, participants can use the G.R.E.E.N. **Action Tracker** sheets to track how many G.R.E.E.N. **Action Reports** they receive. Some guides may say there is not enough time in the day to write and read these notes. However, time spent focusing on this pro-Team behavior can lead to improved Team interactions and help the Team reach its **Common Team Goal**.

G.R.E.E.N. ACTION REPORT

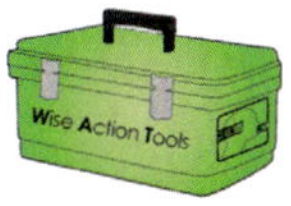

Date: ____________ Situation: ____________

____

____

Who acted G.R.E.E.N.? ____________________

Circle the behavior(s) shown:

Grateful **R**espectful **E**mpathetic **E**asygoing **N**avigating

What was the **G.R.E.E.N.** action? ____________________

____

____

GROWING G.R.E.E.N. InterActions® ©HeinSLP, INC.

Personal G.R.E.E.N. Action Tracker

The **Personal G.R.E.E.N. Action Tracker** (Figure 23) can be filled out daily, giving guides and participants a valuable opportunity to discuss actions that showed they were **Grateful, Respectful, Empathetic, Easygoing,** or **Navigating**. More important than actual totals or worrying about which action goes into which **G.R.E.E.N.** category is supporting the participant's growing desire to engage in prosocial behavior through this process of evaluation and reinforcement of **positive** actions. Participants are given time to review their **G.R.E.E.N. Action Reports** and record their daily numbers on their Personal **G.R.E.E.N. Action Trackers**. This reinforces the growing **positive** participant behavior. Participants can work toward their personal bests, whether displaying increased **G.R.E.E.N.** behavior daily or weekly.

MY NAME ______________________________

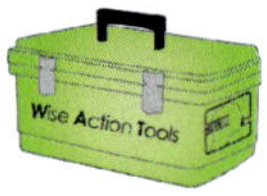

MY PERSONAL G.R.E.E.N. ACTION TRACKER

How many times can I act G.R.E.E.N. this week?

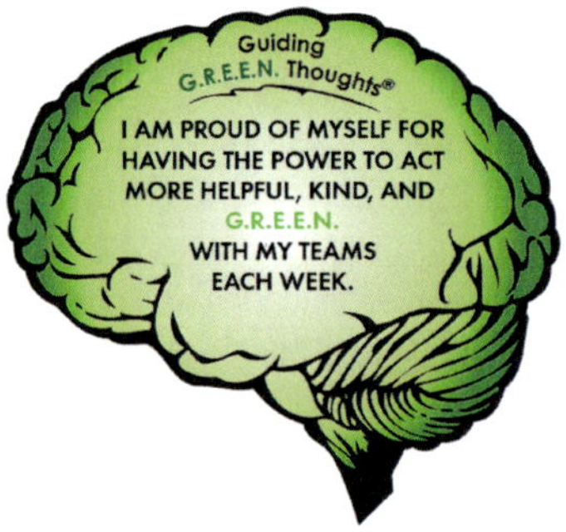

I am acting G.R.E.E.N. when I take action that others think is caring, civil, cooperative, considerate, easygoing, empathetic, grateful, helpful, kind, navigating, polite, positive, respectful, supportive, or thoughtful. When others on my Teams notice me acting G.R.E.E.N. and give me a G.R.E.E.N. Action Report, I put a check mark in the box for that day. I also can fill out a G.R.E.E.N. Action Report for myself when I notice that I have acted G.R.E.E.N.with someone, and I can then give myself a check mark in the box for that day.

I see how many times I can act G.R.E.E.N. this week.
Then I can see if I can act G.R.E.E.N. even more times next week!

Date	Date	Date	Date	Date	Date	Date

This week's G.R.E.E.N. Action Total: ___________

Growing G.R.E.E.N. InterActions® HeinSLP, Inc. www.heinslpinc.com

Figure 23. My Personal G.R.E.E.N. Action Tracker form

Like strengthening a sports-related motor skill by practicing it repeatedly, participant awareness of G.R.E.E.N. behavior is strengthened because it is noticed, described in words, written, reviewed, and then reinforced. Research shows that brain neurons that "fire together, wire together." In other words, the more that brain cells are activated by certain actions, the easier it becomes to engage in these activities the next time.

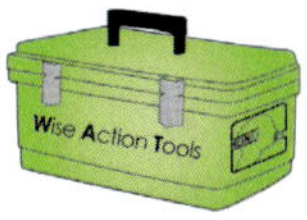

CLASSROOM TEAM G.R.E.E.N. ACTION TRACKER

Name of our Classroom Team: ______________________________

This is our Team Action Tracker for the week starting on ______________
(date)

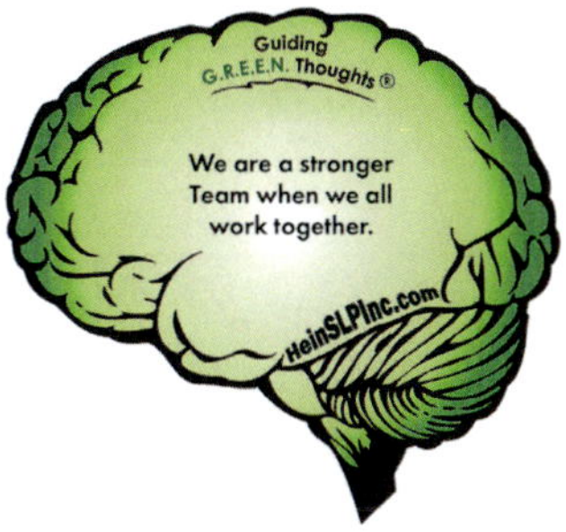

Fill in the names of everyone on the Team.

√ Check the box under the date each time a Classroom Team member acted G.R.E.E.N. or transfer the total from each Team member's **Personal G.R.E.E.N. Action Tracker**.

Classroom Teammates	Monday	Tuesday	Wednesday	Thursday	Friday	Individual Totals

This week's Team total: ____________

Growing G.R.E.E.N. InterActions® HeinSLP, Inc. www.heinslpinc.com

Figure 24. G.R.E.E.N. Action Tracker for the Classroom Team

G.R.E.E.N. Action Tracker for Classroom and Home Teams

So that everyone on the Team sees that they have a place in this Growing G.R.E.E.N. process, G.R.E.E.N. **Action Tracker** charts can be put on the bulletin board for a Classroom Team (Figure 24) or put up on the refrigerator or somewhere else for the Home Team. Everyone is included! Participants appreciate when guides are included on the charts, creating the sense that *we* are all part of the Team. No one is excluded from receiving credit for their G.R.E.E.N. behavior.

Each guide can decide how to reinforce behavior that leads to G.R.E.E.N. actions that help the Team, with reinforcement matching the format of their environment.

One additional tool for reinforcing participant behavior is the G.R.E.E.N. **Certificate** (Figure 25). The certificate can be given to an individual or a whole group at the discretion of the guide. Additional praise may be provided when presenting the certificate.

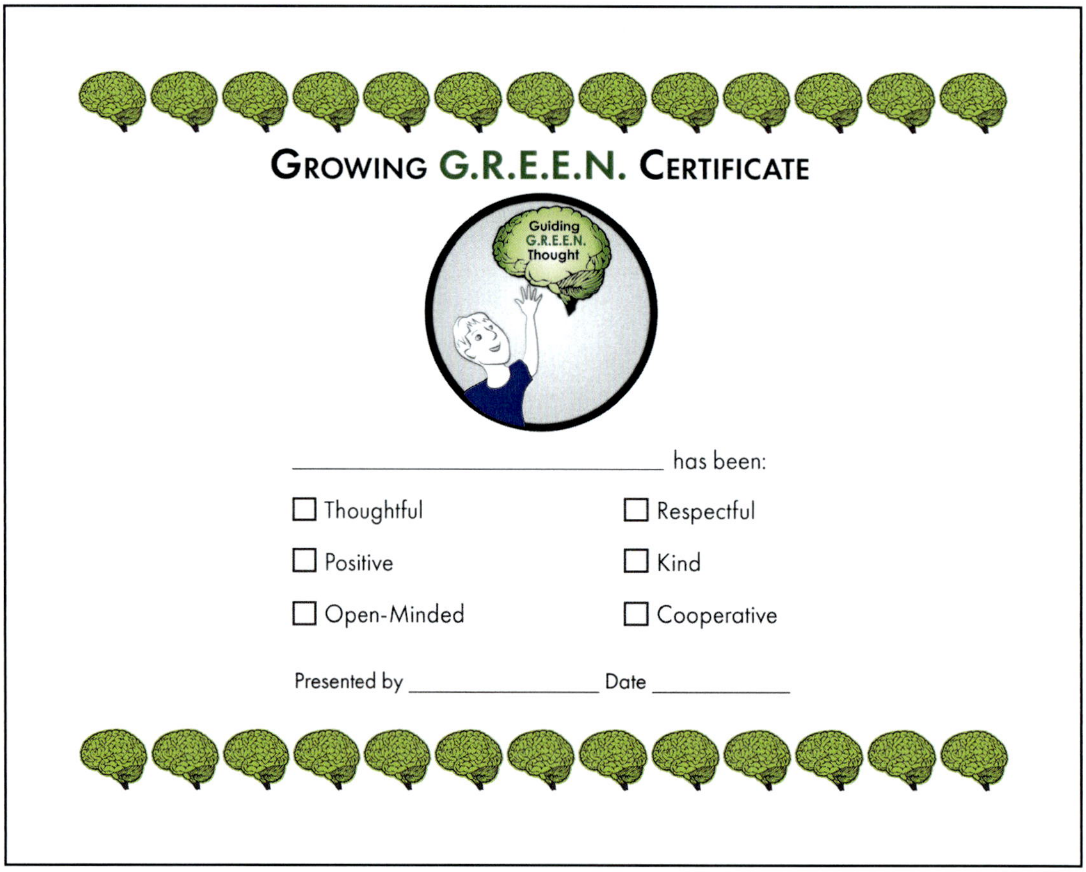

Figure 25. Growing G.R.E.E.N. Certificate

5.10 Guide Participants to Choose and Use Guiding G.R.E.E.N. Thoughts

"She does not have words in her head to guide her actions."

"He just does what he feels like doing impulsively."

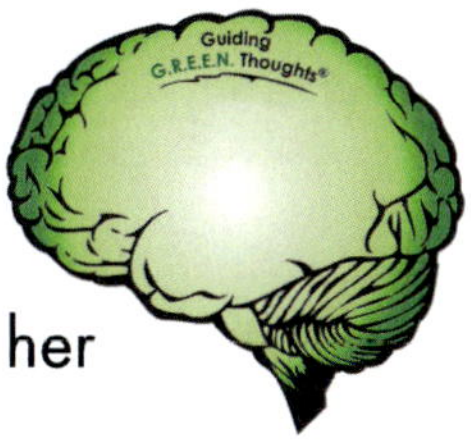

Or "What **Guiding G.R.E.E.N. Thought** can I present to her to guide her best actions now?"

"What **Guiding G.R.E.E.N. Thought** can he choose from to remind him to think before taking action?"

Growing G.R.E.E.N. InterActions introduces unique thoughts and affirmations to guide participants in their thinking and decision-making for varied situations. Based on the participant needs, the guide can select and present appropriate **Guiding G.R.E.E.N. Thoughts**, lessons, and scenes. Participants can be guided to learn the benefits of these thoughts and enjoy acting out related scenes. **Guiding G.R.E.E.N. Thought** cards can be kept in schoolrooms or taken home to support the use of these **Guiding G.R.E.E.N. Thoughts** in real-life scenes outside the classroom. Participants also are encouraged to think of and use their own **Guiding G.R.E.E.N. Thoughts** as long as they benefit the Team. Focusing on the terminology and use of **Guiding G.R.E.E.N. Thoughts** encourages proactive, self-guiding behavior.

5.11 Practice Pathways That Strengthen Targeted Prosocial and New Behavior

"He never remembers how to act."

"She does not say what I told her to say."

Or "He remembers what to say because he practiced this script."

"She has been practicing, and as a result she has improved her skill and confidence."

This program provides many opportunities to practice new ways of analyzing scenes and acting in them. There are new ways to calm oneself down and look at information so it can be analyzed effectively, new scripts to follow for what can be said in different situations, and many other new ways to Think First before interacting. The more the participant is given an opportunity to engage in a new behavior, the stronger the pathways become for new prosocial behavior rather than older, more impulsive, and less social ones.

Participants practice analyzing and **surveying the scene** to determine whether all characters in scenes are helping the Team meet the Common Team Goal. Participants also benefit from multiple opportunities to decide what Personal Goal a character is achieving or striving to achieve. These practice opportunities and related discussions about these kinds of goals can help participants think more frequently about their Personal Goals and Common Team Goals. When role-playing related **G.R.E.E.N. Scenes** on a "movie set," participants are often eager to repeat the scenes to make them even better. Participants practice interacting in prosocial, G.R.E.E.N. ways and begin to feel and enjoy G.R.E.E.N. InterAction success. Concurrently, from these scenes, they learn how to meet the Common Team Goals of Home, School, and Friendship Teams while moving toward meeting Personal Goals. Participants practice seeing themselves as part of the scripted team. This helps the individual work more closely with other people in the scene to achieve the best possible outcome. They practice working together using prosocial, positive, and helpful G.R.E.E.N. InterActions to ensure that Personal and Common Team Goals are met. Participants also frequently practice thinking of **Guiding G.R.E.E.N. Thoughts** to help them achieve mutually beneficial goals. In all of the above, participants practice Thinking First, a critical skill they can carry over to real-life interactions.

5.12 What Is the Main Idea? Helping Students Remember What Is Taught

"This student does not remember anything we talked about."

"This student is not carrying skills and strategies over from one session to the next."

Or ➡ "This student benefits from our taking time together to determine the main idea of this lesson."

➡ "This student remembers what I have been teaching and is using it in other situations."

No matter what is being taught, spending time to clearly spell out the main idea of the lesson can be valuable:

- "This is what we are going to learn about."
- "This is what we are learning now."
- "This is what we learned today. Let's write it down in our lesson log."
- "Let's review what we learned last time."

It is important that the guide and participant state what is learned (Figure 26). This is a good check of participant involvement, with the guide providing as much assistance as needed. By taking the time to "name" the main idea being taught and having the participant "name" it, too, it becomes more likely that the concept, skill, or strategy will be remembered in the next session and in less structured activities.

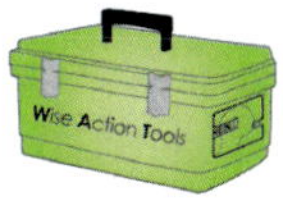

LESSON LOG FOR WHAT I AM LEARNING

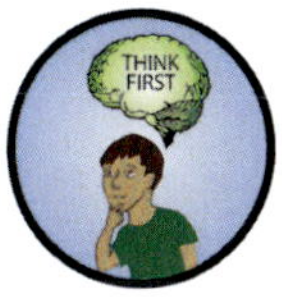

Date	Main Idea of What I Did and Learned Today

Growing G.R.E.E.N. InterActions® HeinSLP, Inc. www.heinslpinc.com

Figure 26. Lesson Log

5.13 Using Music to Encourage and Reinforce G.R.E.E.N. Actions

"We don't have time for music."

Or ➡ "I can see how this music helps us integrate the mood and message of the program."

Guides can make use of another unique aspect of this program—songs that aid in teaching main lessons. Besides being an experienced speech-language pathologist, Herb is a singer-songwriter who has written songs for use in structured lessons. Participants can listen to or sing them whenever they could be beneficial during non-structured activities.

Songs for Guiding G.R.E.E.N. Thoughts (Figure 27) incorporates melodies, lyrics, and instrumentation that help participants engage in the process, and provide an additional modality for teaching the program's main concepts. The songs can be

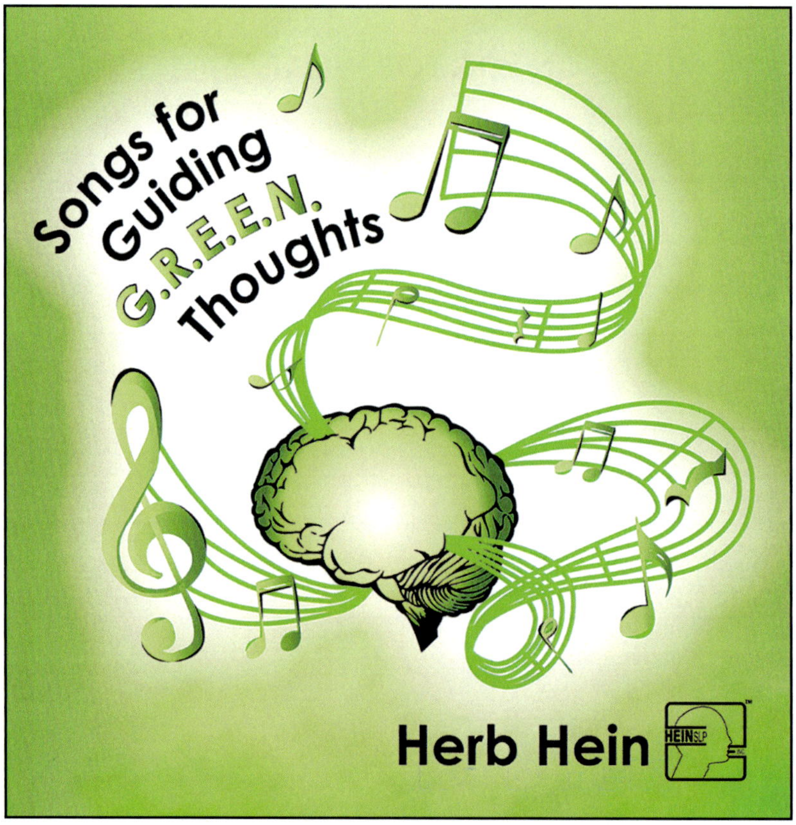

Figure 27. *Songs for Guiding G.R.E.E.N. Thoughts*

played as they appear in the book to signal target behaviors, strategies, and concepts on which to focus. They also can be made available for individual, independent listening with headphones. The songs are self-calming ("Brake to Take a Five Break"), **transformational** ("Keep the **Civil** in **Civil**ization," "**Transformation** Song"), and inspirational for thinking and acting **G.R.E.E.N.** ("Wake Up," "What's Best for the Team," "Guiding **G.R.E.E.N.** Thought Song," "Don't Listen to the Moon," "It's Not All About Me," "Cooperation's in the Air," "You Are a Friend of Mine," "I Don't Ignore You," "I Appreciate").

5.14 Guides As Team Role Models for Acting G.R.E.E.N.

"Do as I say, not as I do."

Or ➡ "I can see that when we all act **G.R.E.E.N.**, our Team becomes even more **powerful**."

Don't forget that you are part of the Team, too. As you teach participants to avoid being impulsive and to be **open-minded** and cooperative, you must act the same way. You are a role model. Monitor yourself to make sure you are being a good role model. Acting like a Team means that everyone on the Team is involved in achieving the **Common Team Goal**. At times, participants have attempted to act as part of a Team only to find that another member of the Team (perhaps even a teacher or parent) has not displayed respectful, cooperative behavior. For this program to make a difference in participant behavior, guides must model **respectful**, **cooperative**, and **collaborative** Team behavior.

5.15 Guides Have More Than One Choice, Too

"We are going to do what I say."

Or ➡ "Let's review our choices to see which is best for all of us."

As guides, we must model flexible thinking. Usually more than one choice must be considered in determining the kind of action to take in a given situation. We should model the procedure of listening to the choices, then making the best choice based on the situation. The procedure and criteria for making choices can be found on the Civilized **Choice Checker** (first introduced as Figure 13):

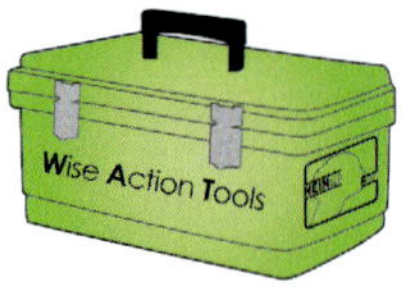

CIVILIZED CHOICE CHECKER

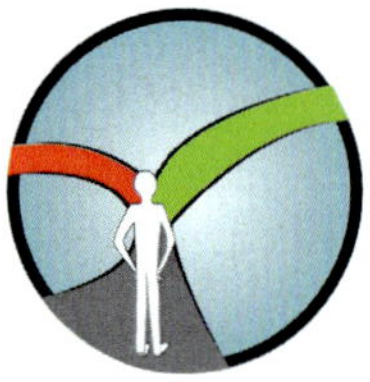

When I **survey this scene**, I think this is happening:

____

This is one way to act **(Choice A)**: ____________________

____

This is another way to act **(Choice B)**: ____________________

____

	Write "+" for **yes** and "-" for **no**	
	Action Choice A	Action Choice B
1. This is a logical choice. Things will get better instead of worse.		
2. This is a safe choice. People will *not* get hurt. Things will *not* get broken.		
3. This choice is good for everyone. Things will be better for *everyone* in the scene.		
4. This choice uses good self-control to meet the goals.		
Total score: Add up the + signs to see which choice is the best. Which choice wins?		

Growing G.R.E.E.N. InterActions ® HeinSLP, Inc. www.heinslpinc.com

We want participants to be open to various choices, so we need to make sure we are open to listening to different choices ourselves. This often involves engaging in a Cooperative Conversation (discussed in Section 4.19) in which the guide models the respectful, collaborative process of full listening, sharing thoughts, and calmly determining, with others, the best actions to take with the Team.

Thank you for taking the time to learn how to be a guide for **Growing G.R.E.E.N. InterActions** with those on your Teams. Here's to us all successfully working together *to be our better selves in a better world!*

Made in United States
Orlando, FL
04 November 2026

90200640R00055